Breast Lu

A Guide to Diseases ui the Breast

Jane Smith, BSc (Hons)
Medical Writer and Editor, Bristol
and
David J. Leaper, MD, ChM, FRCS, FACS
Professor of Surgery, Professorial Unit of Surgery, University Hospital
of North Tees, University of Newcastle upon Tyne, Stockton on Tees

tfm Publishing Limited
Castle Hill Barns
Harley
Nr Shrewsbury
SY5 6LX
UK.

Tel: +44 (0)1952 510061; Fax: +44 (0)1952 510192
E-mail: nikki@tfmpublishing.co.uk; Web site: www.tfmpublishing.co.uk

Design and layout: Nikki Bramhill
Illustrations: Jane Fallows

First published 1994, by Hodder Headline Plc
338 Euston Road, London, NW1 3BH

Second edition
Copyright © J. Smith 2003
ISBN 1 903378 08 7

Printed by Ebenezer Baylis & Son Ltd., The Trinity Press, London Road, Worcester, WR5 2JH, UK.
Tel: +44 (0)1905 357979; Fax: +44 (0)1905 354919.

Contents

Preface to first edition

For many women, the development of any breast abnormality is a cause of fear - the fear of cancer. For 1 in 10 women in the UK who are referred to a specialist because of breast problems, the diagnosis of breast cancer will be the beginning of a difficult and anxious time. Even women with a benign breast disorder may face a series of tests and possibly surgery, and their anxieties should not be overlooked. An understanding of what is likely to happen and why during the process of diagnosis and treatment goes some way towards relieving the anxiety for these women and their families.

Although the relief for a woman who discovers that her condition is benign may be tremendous, she still has a problem that must be dealt with. She may, for example, experience breast pain that makes her life a misery, and it is hoped that this book will be useful for women in this position as well as for those with more serious breast disease.

Breast cancer is not a single entity: there are different types with different prognoses, and a variety of factors - such as whether it has spread to other parts of the body - can affect the outcome.

This book provides details about all the main breast problems and how they can be treated. It also explains what happens before, during and after breast surgery, for both benign and malignant disease, the complications that can occur, and the further treatment and care that may be required for some types of cancer.

The aim of the book is to give women enough practical information to take an active part in the decision-making processes that will affect their own lives.

Jane Smith
David J. Leaper
1994

Preface to second edition

This new edition of *Breast Lumps* (which was first published in 1994) provides updated information on both benign breast conditions and breast cancer. The book has been substantially revised, particularly with regard to the changes that have occurred in the treatment of breast cancer during the last few years. It includes details of the recently introduced guidelines for breast cancer treatment in the UK, and discusses all aspects of the management of breast lumps and the ways in which this differs in the UK and USA.

It is vital that women are involved in the decisions made about their health and therefore that they have access to all the relevant information to help them make the right choices about their own health care. It is hoped that this second edition of *Breast Lumps* will help give women, their families and carers a clear understanding of the various breast conditions and their treatment, and that it will clarify specific aspects they may want to raise with their doctors and/or breast care nurses.

Jane Smith
David J. Leaper
2002

Acknowledgements

Thanks are due to the many people who gave so generously of their time and knowledge in the preparation of this second edition of *Breast Lumps* as well as of the first edition of the book.

We are particularly grateful to Mr Anthony Peel, Consultant Surgeon (retired), University Hospital of North Tees, Stockton on Tees, Specialist in Breast and Upper Gastrointestinal Surgery; Mr John Kenealy, Plastic and Reconstructive Surgeon at Frenchay Hospital, Bristol; Dr John Graham, Consultant in Clinical Oncology at the Bristol Oncology Centre; Dr Elisabeth Kutt, Consultant Radiologist at the Avon Breast Screening Clinic, Bristol; Dr Alasdair Dow, Consultant in Anaesthesia and Intensive Care at the Royal Devon and Exeter Hospital; Jane Barker, Clinical Nurse Specialist, North Bristol NHS Trust, Frenchay Hospital, Bristol; and to Dr Suzanne Klimberg, Professor of Surgery and Pathology and Director of the Division of Breast Surgical Oncology, of the Breast Cancer Program and of the Breast Fellowship in Diseases of the Breast at the University of Arkansas for Medical Sciences, and Staff Physician at the Central Arkansas Veterans Healthcare System, Little Rock, Arkansas, USA, for her perspective on treatment in the USA.

We are also grateful for the help given in the preparation of the first edition by Dr Ian Donaldson, GP; Gill Down, Clinical Nurse Specialist at Southmead Hospital, Bristol; Judy Vickery (Ward Sister), Hazel Elliott (Clinical Nurse Specialist in Palliative Care), and Caroline Cree (Superintendent Physiotherapist), at Southmead Hospital, Bristol; Mrs Rose West and the staff of The BUPA Hospital Bristol; Mr John Loosley of the Bristol and District Community Health Council; and Jo Hudson, Clinical Nurse Specialist at the Bristol Oncology Centre.

Chapter 1

Introduction

Pain and lumps in the breast can have various causes and most are due to non-malignant (benign) disorders that are not life threatening, although some can result in considerable discomfort. In fact, more than 90% of women who are referred to a specialist with breast symptoms have benign conditions, the majority of which can usually be effectively treated.

This book deals with the more common non-malignant breast conditions as well as with the various types of breast cancer that can develop in women. (Although diseases of the breast do occur in men, they are much less common and are not dealt with here.)

Before looking at the different breast disorders and their causes, it is helpful to understand the meaning of some of the key words that are used in this book and that may be used by your doctor, and to have some knowledge of the structure of the breast and its development.

❖ A **cancer** is a growth caused by the uncontrolled multiplication of cells. If left untreated, it will eventually invade nearby areas of the body and spread to more distant parts.

❖ A **tumour** is a swelling, which may or may not be cancerous. It is a non-specific term that can cause confusion.

❖ **Benign** (or **non-malignant**) describes a disease or condition from which complete recovery is likely following adequate treatment. **Benign tumours** remain localized at the site at which they develop (i.e. they do not spread). They have no harmful effect other than possibly to press on nearby organs, thus interfering with their normal function.

❖ **Malignant** (or **cancerous**) describes a disease or condition that is likely to spread locally and, in most cases, to distant parts of the body. **Malignant tumours** invade the surrounding tissue, and their cells may eventually be carried to other body organs, where they develop into secondary tumours called **metastases**.

❖ The process of spread of cancer cells is called **metastasis**.

❖ **Pre-malignant** refers to a disease or condition that has the *potential* to become cancerous.

❖ **Lymph** is a pale-coloured fluid containing disease-fighting cells called **lymphocytes**. It flows around the body within the **lymphatic vessels**. Cancer cells can be spread to other parts of the body within the lymphatic system.

❖ **Lymph nodes** are glands into which the lymphatic vessels drain. The presence of cancer cells in the lymph nodes is a sign that the cancer is spreading.

❖ A **palpable** lump is one that can be felt by touch.

❖ A **non-palpable** lump cannot be felt.

Structure and function of the breast

The breast is a gland (the mammary gland), which is made up of several lobules of glandular tissue, separated by fibrous material. It is embedded in fat, which gives it its smooth surface and most of its bulk.

The function of the breasts in all female mammals is to produce milk for the developing young. Milk production occurs in the lobules of the breast and the milk passes via lactiferous ducts to the nipple. Around each nipple is a pigmented area called the areola, which is lubricated by oily secretions from sebaceous glands in the skin.

Blood is taken to and from the breast through numerous arteries and veins. There is also a system of lymph vessels that drain lymph from the surface to deep within the breast, and from there to lymph nodes mostly in the armpit (axilla), and in the chest wall adjacent to the collarbone (clavicle), and the breast-bone (sternum).

The lymphatic drainage of the breast is particularly important in malignant disease because cancer cells are able to spread via the lymph

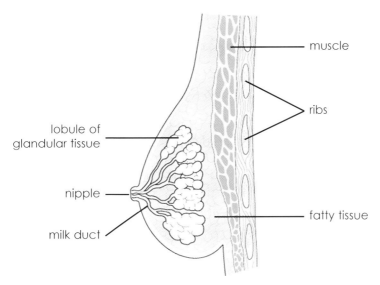

muscle

ribs

lobule of
glandular tissue

nipple

fatty tissue

milk duct

The female breast.

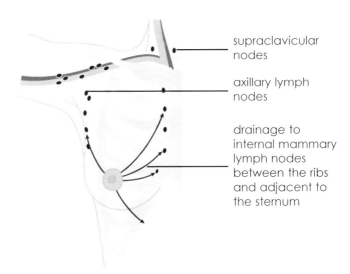

supraclavicular
nodes

axillary lymph
nodes

drainage to
internal mammary
lymph nodes
between the ribs
and adjacent to
the sternum

Lymphatic drainage from the breast. *The arrows indicate the main pathways of drainage of lymph from the breast to the surrounding lymph nodes.*

vessels to other areas of the body, particularly to the axillary lymph nodes of the armpit. However, swollen, inflamed (non-malignant) lymph nodes can also develop in benign conditions.

Development of the breast

As a fetus develops in the womb, part of its chest wall turns inwards to form a series of branching ducts. Just before birth, the ducts turn out again, forming the nipple. In girls at puberty, many small, sac-like alveoli sprout from the ends of the ducts and fat is laid down around them. The glandular alveoli develop further during pregnancy and secrete droplets of milk in lactation.

In general, as women get older, the gland tissue in their breasts is gradually replaced by fat, which is why the breasts become softer and tend to droop with age. Eventually, most of the ducts and lobules disappear.

Tender nodules may appear as the breasts begin to develop at puberty and this tenderness may remain for months or even years. Once the breasts have developed, any pain or lump that forms needs to be investigated. Early detection and removal of a small cancerous breast lump probably give a better chance of cure and survival - and of saving the breast - than treatment of a larger lump that has begun to spread to other parts of the body.

Details of some of the most common benign breast disorders and of the different types of breast cancer are given in Chapters 5 and 6, respectively.

A poorly fitting bra can cause breast pain

If you develop breast pain for which there is no obvious cause and you cannot detect any swelling in the breast, it may first be worth checking that you are wearing a correctly fitting bra. If you gain or lose weight, you will need to wear a larger or smaller bra than previously, but many women continue to wear the same size for years, despite weight fluctuations. Specialists often see women whose bras are too small or too large and are causing them considerable discomfort and/or failing to provide support for their breasts.

Good lingerie departments in large department stores and specialist shops have trained staff to measure women for the right size of bra, and many of these assistants also have experience in helping women to find well-fitting bras following breast surgery. Bras of sizes outside the normal manufactured range that cannot be ordered by shops can be specially made. A breast care nurse, consultant or someone in the appliance department at your local hospital should be able to give you advice and information about where to obtain these.

How to measure yourself for a bra

It is quite simple to measure yourself for a bra if you prefer not to be measured by someone else, or if you want to check that the bra you are wearing is right for you.

- *For bra size.* With your bra removed, measure around your back and across your ribs, with the tape measure passing under your bust. If the measurement *in inches* is an even number, add 4 to obtain your bra size. If the measurement in inches is uneven, add 5. For example:

  actual measurement = 31 inches
  add 5 (as this is an uneven number) = 36. (1)
  Therefore, your correct bra size is 36 inches.

- *For cup size.* Measure from the centre of your spine, under your arm and across the fullest part of one breast to the bone between your breasts. This gives a more accurate figure than measuring around your back and across both breasts. (You may need to ask someone to do this for you.) Double the number of *inches* obtained to give the full measurement. Then take away your bra size (measurement (1) above) and use your answer and the chart below to find your cup size. For example:

  measurement of half body = 20 inches
  double this (20 x 2) = 40 inches
  subtract bra size (36 in this example) = 40-36 = 4 inches. (2)

Chart of cup sizes

1 inch	A
2 inches	B
3 inches	C
4 inches	D

Therefore, in this example, the correct bra size is 36D.

This method is useful as a guide when buying a bra, but sizes vary slightly amongst the different manufacturers and the only way to be sure you get a well-fitting bra is to try some on.

Chapter 2

Breast examination

Although in most cases breast lumps and pain are due to benign conditions, it is advisable to see your doctor as soon as possible if you notice any change in your breasts. The early detection and treatment of breast cancer could mean having an operation to remove a small lump, which leaves a small scar, rather than losing a breast altogether. Even more importantly, it could save your life.

Signs of disease

There are various signs of disease that a doctor will look for, some of which you may be able to detect yourself by regularly examining your breasts (see below). These signs include:

❖ a newly apparent lump that is persistent rather than cyclical (i.e. that is not related to your menstrual cycle),

❖ reddening of the skin (indicating inflammation),

❖ obvious veins that are more visible on one side of the breast,

❖ a change in the general shape of the breast,

❖ dimpling of the skin of the breast,

❖ a retracted or weeping nipple,

❖ a swollen node in the neck or under the arm.

Although nipple discharge can be associated with various diseases, it may also be an early sign of a cancer (particularly if bloody) and can occur before any lump is large enough to be felt.

A malignant tumour that is close to the surface of the breast may pull at the overlying skin, causing it to dimple slightly. Another serious sign is a condition known as *peau d'orange*, in which the skin of the breast becomes pitted like that of an orange. It occurs because the lymph vessels (which drain fluid away from the breast) become blocked and the breast swells as the fluid accumulates. The tiny pits are due to tethering of small areas of the skin between the lymphatic swellings.

Ulceration of a cancer through the skin is a late sign of advanced disease, although, paradoxically, it is not necessarily a sign of a poor outcome.

Breast awareness

Most of the signs of disease mentioned above can only be detected by looking at the breasts. It is therefore now generally accepted that being aware of the normal appearance of your breasts and regularly inspecting them for any apparent changes may be more important than breast self-examination that is done by feeling them - known as palpation.

If you are confident about examining your breasts by touch, you should continue to do this, but it is important that you also look at them and are aware of any visible abnormal changes that occur. If you do not like feeling your breasts yourself, simply being aware of any change in their appearance or an abnormal sensation is a reasonable alternative, although you can ask your family doctor or practice nurse to check them for you.

Practising breast awareness from the time the breasts develop may be beneficial and can be done, for example, while applying deodorant with your arm raised, or in the bath or shower.

Breast self-examination

Examination of the breasts needs to be done regularly and properly to be useful. Once a month is probably ideal, a few days after a period when the breasts are least 'active'. Some women find self-examination a source of considerable anxiety, or they worry because they do not do it. Very often, women who do discover a lump or any other abnormality in their breasts are slow to report it to their doctors. Their fear is understandable, but usually unjustified. The lumps detected by approximately 8-9 out of every 10 women turn out to be benign.

Although there is some controversy about whether or not the early detection of small, cancerous lumps by breast self-examination has any significant effect on the outcome of treatment, the results of several studies suggest that it might do so. Breast self-examination is now generally accepted as being a useful and positive way in which women can help to monitor their own health.

As women age, the amount of fat in their breasts increases, and older women, as well as those who are overweight or who have very large breasts, may find it more difficult to distinguish between normal and abnormal changes when they feel their breasts.

If you are unable to examine your breasts for any reason, it may be possible for this to be done by your doctor or by a specially trained nurse. However, it is more useful for you to 'get to know' your own breasts and therefore to be able to detect any changes that occur in the breast tissue.

When to do it

Monthly examinations should be carried out a few days after the start of each menstrual period, because the breasts tend to be tender and lumpy before and during the period, making assessment more difficult. If you do not have periods, you should examine your breasts on the same day of each month.

How to do it

Although the following is a description of the ideal method of breast examination, some women prefer to examine their breasts in the shower, and this is certainly better than not doing it at all.

Examining your breasts

To examine your breasts, first remove all the clothing from the top half of your body and stand in front of a mirror. Look at the whole of each breast, turning sideways as you do so. Then raise your arms above your head and look again, especially at the area around the nipple. Look for any signs of tethering of the skin. If you know your body well, you should be able to detect anything unusual, i.e. anything that is a change from what is normal for you. Make sure you become familiar with the normal size, shape and general appearance of your breasts and nipples.

Next, put your hands on your hips and press inwards until the muscles in your chest become tense. If the skin over a breast seems to pit or dimple, if a breast changes shape, or if the nipples of the two breasts do not point the same way, you should make an appointment for your doctor to examine you. Also check your nipples for any discharge, as this may be a sign of a minor or more serious problem. Any flaky rash or change in the appearance of the nipple, particularly with reduction of the projection or weeping of the skin, should be taken very seriously and should be reported to your general practitioner.

Then continue your examination by lying on your back on a bed with your head on a pillow. To examine your left breast, put a folded towel under your left shoulder and use the flat part of the fingers of your right hand (not the fingertips) to feel the breast. Keeping your fingers together, press your breast firmly but gently all over. Start by working in a circular pattern around the nipple and continue outwards. Then, raising your left arm above your head, continue to examine up towards and into your armpit.

Repeat the whole process for your right breast, with the towel under your right shoulder and feeling with the fingers of your left hand.

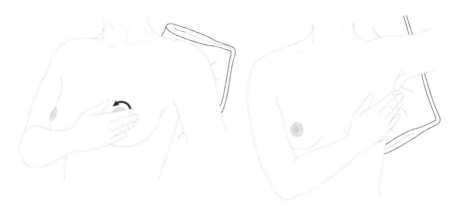

Breast self-examination. *(See text for details.)*

Signs to look for

When you have completed your examinations, consider the following questions.

❖ Has either of your breasts changed in size?

❖ Has there been a change in, or is there a discharge or bleeding from, a nipple?

❖ Is there unusual pitting or dimpling of the skin of the breast or of the nipple?

❖ Can you feel a lump or thickening within the breast? The normal breast is firm but may contain lumps, which are often most prominent just before a period. If you can feel an unusual lump, is it hard or soft, regular or irregular in shape?

If you do detect any change, or are concerned for any reason, make an appointment to see your doctor.

If you examine your breasts regularly, either by palpation (touch) or by looking at them, you will get to know their normal feel and appearance and should be better able to detect any change that may occur. It is also a good idea to get into the habit of checking your breasts when you are showering, for example, rather than just when you are carrying out breast self-examination.

Chapter 3

Diagnostic investigations

If you visit your family doctor because you have pain in your breast or have detected a breast lump, you will probably be referred to a breast clinic for further investigations. Specialists in breast cancer have more experience of treating women with breast disease than surgeons who also deal with a variety of other conditions. It is therefore wise for all women to see a breast specialist. Breast specialists also have a full 'support team', including nurse counsellors, and meet regularly with other specialists to decide on the best treatment for their patients. These multidisciplinary meetings involve surgeons, nurse breast specialists (breast care nurses), radiologists, pathologists and oncologists and, in the UK, are run on nationally agreed guidelines.

If your doctor suspects that you may have breast cancer, he or she will write a letter or send a fax to a breast clinic asking for an appointment to be made for you to have an assessment. As a result of a recent National Health Service (NHS) directive in the UK, all women with suspected breast cancer must be offered an appointment within 2 weeks of referral. If cancer is diagnosed, or suspected, the course of events may vary slightly from that described below, depending on the normal procedure at your particular hospital.

If, having seen a breast specialist, you would like a second opinion, do discuss this with your doctor, the practice nurse or the hospital breast care nurse. You should be able to choose to be treated elsewhere if you have any concerns about the treatment you are being offered, but, in practice, you may have to be prepared to push hard to get what you want.

Clinic visits

The one-stop clinic

There are now one-stop clinics in most areas in the UK, which combine clinical assessment, imaging (see p.14) and, where appropriate, aspiration cytology (see p. 18). This combined process is known as triple assessment and is mandatory for women over the age of 35 with breast problems, but cannot always be provided for women under this age.

❖ For *women aged over 35*, the initial assessment is made with the imaging process known as mammography (see p.14). If the mammogram shows a suspicious area of your breast, you will then have magnification mammography, ultrasound and cytology. Before examining your breasts, the clinician will take a full history, including any details of relevant family history, menstrual status and any previous breast problems. Despite the introduction of the various imaging techniques, breast examination has not been rendered obsolete, because not all breast pathology is detectable on mammography.

❖ *Women aged less than 35* will also be seen for assessment as soon as possible, within 2 weeks if their doctor suspects breast cancer, but certainly within 3-4 weeks. At the clinic, a full medical history will be taken and your breasts will be examined before arrangements are made for imaging. Cytology may also be done at this time, although it can cause bruising, which makes interpretation of the subsequent imaging more difficult. Ultrasound (see p.17) will be done if there are suspicious findings or if there is an irregular lump.

Mammography may also be of value for women between the ages of 30 and 35, particularly for those who have had children and who have breast-fed. It is less useful for younger women because their breast tissue is very dense.

Family history clinics

Many breast units have family history clinics for women with a first-degree relative (e.g. sister or mother) who developed breast cancer before the age of 50. If you have an affected first-degree relative, you may be offered regular mammography, which should start 5 years before the age at which your relative developed breast cancer, or when you are aged 35.

Some specialists prefer to discuss at the first clinic visit the possible courses of action that could be taken if cancer is confirmed. They feel this allows women time to consider their options and to talk things over with their families. Other specialists prefer to leave any detailed discussions until a second clinic visit when the results of the tests are known. You may wish to consider for yourself which option you would prefer, so that you are ready to ask the specialist to discuss things with you at the outset if you feel this would be helpful.

Always remember that you are free to do nothing: having no treatment is also an option open to you. However, if you are considering this option, you should talk it over carefully with your specialist or breast care nurse, as it may severely reduce your chances of survival if you have breast cancer or may result in you suffering unnecessary pain and discomfort with other types of breast condition.

For the majority of women, the clinical examination will indicate a benign condition such as a non-malignant tumour, a cyst or a normal change in the breast (see Chapter 5). If further investigations are required, arrangements will be made for these to be carried out.

It is a good idea to take someone with you when you go for your clinic visits, for example your husband, partner or a friend, as it is often difficult to absorb what you are told when you are anxious, particularly if the news is not good. It may also be helpful to have made notes of any questions you want to ask the specialist or breast care nurse (see p. 21).

Investigations

There are various investigations that can be carried out at a hospital or special clinic. The information given here is meant as a guide to what may happen; your own experiences may vary slightly in detail from what is described.

Mammography

Mammography involves taking X-rays of the soft tissues of the breast and armpit. It is used for routine breast screening (see Chapter 4) and as a tool in the diagnosis of breast diseases.

The natural contrast due to the breast's fat content is exploited in mammography. Most breast cancers occur in women over the age of 45, and it is around this age that glandular tissue within the breast begins to be replaced by fat. As different types of growth vary in appearance, quite accurate distinction can be made between some benign and malignant lumps.

Young women who are concerned about breast cancer (perhaps because they have a family history of the disease) and request a mammogram may find that their request is refused; some then arrange for mammography to be carried out at a private clinic. However, mammograms are not normally helpful in women under the age of 35 because their breast tissue is too dense for most abnormalities to be visible.

Seen on an X-ray, benign breast tumours and cysts (see p. 31) tend to have a smooth outline, sometimes surrounded by a 'halo' of fat. Malignant tumours, on the other hand, are usually poorly defined, more diffuse masses with tendrils extending into the surrounding tissue. Both types of tumour can contain calcium deposits called microcalcifications, the appearance of which can be quite distinctive in different types of breast lumps. In malignant lumps, there are often numerous microcalcifications arranged in lines, suggesting they are running along ducts. This is typical of ductal cancer (see p. 44). By comparison, the microcalcifications in benign breast lumps tend to be much denser and longer, and may look like tea leaves in a teacup. These are sometimes deposits of calcium from an absorbing cyst.

If mammography reveals a lump in your breast, you may have further investigations such as a biopsy (see below).

When is mammography necessary?
Apart from its use as a screening tool for older women (over the age of 50 in the UK and recommended for women over the age of 40 in the USA) and for those who are particularly at risk of developing breast cancer, mammography is important in the diagnosis of various breast diseases. The following are some signs and symptoms that may need to be investigated by mammography:

❖ a lump of unknown origin,

❖ several small lumps that can be felt within the breast,

❖ unexplained discharge from the nipple,

❖ unexplained inversion of the nipple.

When malignant disease is suspected, mammography is also used to:

❖ confirm the clinical diagnosis,

❖ determine the extent of the disease - there may be more than one cancer in the breast,

❖ look for disease that cannot be felt but that may be apparent on a mammogram as areas of calcification,

❖ look for cancer in the other breast.

Mammography can also help in the planning of surgery and to look for signs of recurrent disease or further breast lumps following cancer treatment.

The process of mammography

You will be asked to remove your clothing down to your waist and a radiographer will then help to position you for the X-ray. One of your breasts will be placed on a shelf-like plate on the mammography machine and another plate will be lowered onto the breast to compress it. You will be asked to keep very still while the X-ray is taken. The process will then be repeated for the other breast.

The pressure on the breast as it is compressed between the two plates can be quite uncomfortable, but lasts only a few seconds. Many women are anxious about having a mammogram and so are more than usually sensitive to any discomfort it causes. Some do find the process painful - particularly just before a period - and, rarely, it can cause bruising of the breast, or pain, that can last for several days or weeks. However, the pressure of the plates is unlikely to cause any harm and the radiation level

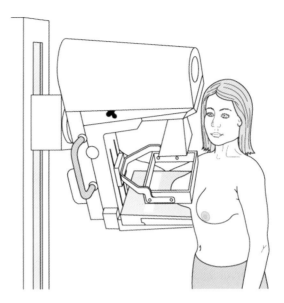

Mammography. *Each breast is compressed between the two plates on the mammography machine while an X-ray is taken.*

from the X-ray is very low (no more than you might be subjected to, for example, during a plane journey). Higher radiation doses are required to take X-rays of the breasts of young women, which is another reason why young women should not have more mammograms than necessary. The benefits of mammography as a diagnostic tool and for breast screening do outweigh any discomfort it may cause.

Ultrasonography

Ultrasonography - also known as ultrasound - is another imaging technique, which, instead of using X-rays, involves passing high-frequency sound waves into the breast. (The process is similar to the sonar system used to detect objects underwater, such as by submarines, and is also used for fetal scanning in pregnant women.) When the sound waves meet a solid object within the breast, they are reflected back like an echo and processed by a computer, which builds up a picture that can be displayed on a screen. This picture is then interpreted by someone trained in ultrasonography and will show the normal glandular tissue and fat quite clearly, as well as any prominent ducts, cysts and tumours.

Ultrasound is particularly useful to distinguish between fluid-filled cysts and solid lumps and, ideally, should be used with mammography and fine-needle aspiration (see below).

Biopsy

Until recently, the diagnosis of breast lumps often involved the surgical removal of a small piece of tissue - called a biopsy. Although this is occasionally still necessary, there are now other techniques that can normally be used instead that do not require a general anaesthetic and can often be done by a surgeon in an out-patients' clinic.

Fine-needle aspiration biopsy

Fine-needle aspiration is a cytological examination (i.e. it involves the study of cells) that can help to confirm the diagnosis of a non-malignant tumour or cyst as well as to detect the presence of cancer cells. It is rare for a cancer to be missed using this technique. However, although it can confirm that a suspicious lump is a cancer, a negative result does not necessarily mean that it is not: the needle may have been inserted into normal tissue around a malignant tumour. Therefore, further tests may be done to confirm a negative result.

Your skin will be wiped with an alcohol wipe before a fine needle is inserted through it. (The needle is about the same size as that used to take blood from the arm.) The surgeon will hold the lump firmly between his or her fingers, push the needle into it several times and draw up a few cells into a syringe. The sample of cells will then be spread on a glass slide, which will be sent to the laboratory to be examined under a microscope. Sometimes, suspicious fluid that has been drawn out of a cyst is also sent to the laboratory in a bottle.

You will be asked to press on the area once the needle has been withdrawn. This is simply to try to limit the amount of bruising that will probably develop, which may last for several days or more. Because of the swelling and bruising that result from needle biopsies, which may make palpation of the breast difficult and a mammogram unclear, it is better if these are not done by a family doctor before a breast clinic visit.

Although a small number of women find the procedure painful, it is usually only uncomfortable. Anaesthetic can only be used to numb the skin for needle aspiration, because it could damage the cells within the breast that are needed for the cytologist to make a diagnosis.

A non-palpable breast lump (i.e. one that cannot be felt) can be located by ultrasound or by mammography using a special mammographic attachment to guide the needle into the lump.

Core biopsy

A core biopsy is a histological examination (i.e. it involves the study of a small sample of solid tissue). The needle used to extract the tissue sample is wider than that used for fine-needle aspiration and has another needle inside it. Local anaesthetic *is* usually used for this procedure, a small amount being injected into the skin over the site of the suspicious lump before the biopsy needle is inserted. A long, very thin core of tissue is removed as the needle is withdrawn, and this is then sent to the laboratory to be examined under a microscope. The process may be repeated several times.

Core biopsies are now commonly carried out in surgical clinics and screening centres and can be useful when a fine-needle aspiration biopsy has failed to provide a definite diagnosis of a palpable lump. Better core biopsy guns have been developed over the last few years, which are guided by ultrasound or X-ray and which can take several samples of tissue (cores) from the breast. These have resulted in more accurate diagnosis and more accurate determination of the tumour type, characteristics, grade etc. They can also be used to assess the body's hormone status, which is useful when deciding whether hormone therapy (see p. 101) is likely to be effective.

Stereotactic core biopsy A modification of the core biopsy technique involves the use of a needle called a Mammotome®, which has a vacuum device attached to it. This technique - called stereotactic core biopsy - enables non-palpable breast lumps (i.e. lumps that cannot be felt) to be located with considerable accuracy and allows several cores of tissue to be sampled through a small incision made in the breast.

During the procedure, you will lie face down on a special table, with your breast protruding through a hole. Your breast will be lightly compressed and a mammography image will be obtained and processed by a computer to pinpoint the site of the lump. The Mammotome® needle will then be guided to the correct position by a computerized system, a small cut will be made in your breast and a single sample containing 6-12 cores of tissue will be removed. The sample will then be X-rayed to make sure it contains the tissue of interest and the small incision in your breast will be closed with a Steri-strip.

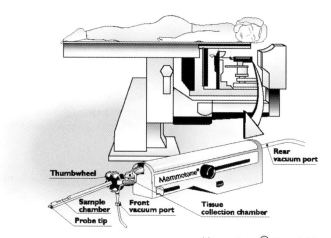

Mammotome® Breast Biopsy System

Stereotactic core biopsy. *A non-palpable lump is located using mammography. A small cut is then made in the breast and a Mammotome® needle is inserted into the lump to remove a sample of several thin cores of tissue.*

This technique has been shown to improve the accuracy of sampling of very small lesions and the vacuum device ensures that bleeding is kept to a minimum.

Tru-Cut® biopsy Before core biopsy guns became widely available, a process called Tru-Cut® biopsy was commonly used. Tru-Cut® biopsies are quite accurate, show the architecture of the breast and aid in the specific typing of cancers, but it is possible for them to miss the appropriate part of the lump because the tissue sample can only be taken from one site. Their use has therefore largely been superseded by that of the newer biopsy techniques.

Grading

Cancers are graded according to the appearance of their cells under a microscope. The grade of a breast cancer gives an indication of how aggressive it is and of how likely it is to spread. Confusingly for patients, there are several different grading systems in use, but, very simply, breast cancers can be divided as follows.

❖ In low-grade (grade I, well-differentiated) breast cancers, the cancer cells appear similar to normal breast cells, with only slight abnormalities.

❖ Intermediate-grade (grade II) breast cancers are moderately differentiated.

❖ High-grade (grade III, poorly differentiated) breast cancers contain cells that appear very abnormal and are quite different from normal breast tissue.

The breast care nurse

Once you have discussed the diagnosis and possible treatment with the specialist, you may wish to talk to a breast care nurse, perhaps to clarify any points you have not understood. At some hospitals, a breast care nurse always attends the clinics; at others, you may be given a card with her name and a contact number. You and your relatives may find it easier to discuss things with a specialist nurse and she will probably be very aware of the worries you are likely to have. Talking things over with a breast care nurse can help you make decisions about your treatment if you have been given a choice of options.

Asking questions

Always ask questions if you are unsure about anything. It is a good idea to write your questions down before your clinic visit, as everyone is apt to forget things in this sort of situation, particularly when they are anxious or nervous.

Never feel embarrassed about the questions you want to ask and never go away not having understood something; it will only cause you to worry. Almost all your questions can be easily answered with simple explanations, but, when this is not possible, your doctor should be able to discuss the reasons with you. Uncertainty and confusion cause anxiety, which, in most cases, is unfounded. If there are still things you are uncertain about once you have left the clinic, contact your breast care nurse, who will be able to discuss these with you.

Being told you have breast cancer

Do not be afraid to speak openly to your doctor. Some doctors avoid mentioning the word 'cancer' and feel the need to shield patients from any unpleasant truths. Some will not explain your diagnosis fully unless you ask them to, believing that you would ask if you wanted to know. Most breast care nurses have had the experience of talking to women who, having been told their diagnosis by a specialist, express relief at discovering that they have a 'tumour and not cancer'. Although a tumour is strictly an abnormal swelling, some doctors use the word when they actually mean a malignant tumour - a cancer. If you are anxious about a lump or do not understand what you are being told about it, it is best to be frank: 'Is it cancer, doctor?' should elicit a direct and truthful answer, although it is a question many people will find difficult to ask.

If you have been told that you have breast cancer, you will need - and should expect - to talk to a breast care nurse. It is easier to come to terms with this disease if you have been given accurate information by a sympathetic, informed professional. All specialist breast units have comprehensive follow-up care, and help and counselling for women with breast cancer and for their families are also available from a variety of organizations. Your breast care nurse, family doctor or consultant will be able to give you information about these services. (See also Appendix IV for some useful addresses.) Most centres also supply information packs for their patients and have details of support groups and volunteers.

Chapter 4

Breast screening

It is known that the incidence of breast cancer increases with age. It is now also generally accepted that the early detection of breast cancer by screening and the accurate diagnosis and treatment of small lumps can improve the outcome in many cases. A study in the USA carried out several years ago found that 95% of women whose breast lumps were detected and treated when measuring 0.5 cm or less in diameter were alive and disease free after 20 years; 70% of women whose breast lumps measured 2-3 cm when detected and treated were alive after 5 years. One Swedish study suggested that regular screening for breast cancer could reduce the mortality rate by as much as 50%.

As a result, since 1989, there has been a national breast-screening programme in the UK that invites women aged between 50 and 65 to undergo mammography every 3 years. There are plans to increase the age of the cut-off point to 70 by the year 2004, but, until then, you may continue to be screened after the age of 65 if you wish to do so, and your local screening centre, family doctor or, currently, a Community Health Council will be able to give you advice about how to arrange this. Currently, about 80% of women in the UK take up the invitation to undergo regular screening, and breast cancer is detected in about 5 in 1000 of them. Although there is no national basis for breast screening in the USA, the American Cancer Society recommends that women over the age of 40 should be screened yearly.

Invitation to attend for breast screening

In the UK, you will receive a letter (and probably an explanatory leaflet) some time after your fiftieth birthday asking you to attend a breast-screening clinic. Most clinics deal with all the patients on the lists of general practitioners in their area at a time, working their way around all the doctors' practices in what is likely to be a programme involving many thousands of women. Because of the numbers involved, some women are not contacted until they are almost 53 years old. However, if you have any particular cause for concern, or think you may have been accidentally omitted from a screening programme, do contact your doctor for advice.

You may be asked to attend a special breast-screening clinic or the mammography department of a hospital. Some clinics also have mobile units that remain in a particular area for a few months, which are convenient for women who do not live close to a clinic or hospital.

First appointment

When you arrive at the clinic, you will be asked a few general questions about your health and then shown into a cubicle to undress to the waist. It is easier if you wear trousers or a skirt rather than a dress. An X-ray of each of your breasts will then be taken, as described on p. 14. You should tell the radiographer if you are concerned about a lump so that you can be recalled for a clinical examination even if your mammogram does not show any abnormality.

Once both breasts have been X-rayed, you will be able to get dressed while you wait a few minutes for the films to be developed and for the radiographer to make sure that they are technically adequate. If you are asked to have a repeat X-ray at this stage, it will be for technical reasons or because a clear picture of the whole area of interest has not been obtained. The radiographer will not have made any medical judgement of your X-rays - only a technical one.

Receiving the results

During the next couple of weeks you and/or your family doctor should receive one of the following letters.

❖ You are likely to receive a letter telling you that the mammogram showed no abnormality and that you will be called again for screening in 3 years' time. This may be phrased as 'no significant abnormality' to take account of the fact that there is no real 'normal' standard because all women's breasts are different.

❖ You may receive a letter asking you to return for another mammogram because your X-rays were technically of poor quality. This may be because you moved slightly while the X-ray was being taken or the developed film may not show enough of the breast area and armpit.

❖ You may receive a letter asking you to return to the clinic for another assessment. This is the case for about 1 woman in 14 and can be because the X-rayed area needs to be examined more closely. Although you are bound to feel concern if this happens, bear in mind that there are numerous changes that occur in the breast tissue with age, some of which are quite normal and some of which may seem abnormal but are harmless.

Of the women who are recalled for further breast screening, 9 out of 10 are found *not* to have cancer. Most of the breast changes apparent on mammograms are not associated with any form of malignancy. Because of the importance of the early detection of breast cancer for successful treatment, the doctor examining your X-rays will err on the side of caution, and any unusual change in the tissue or sign of breast disease will be examined further.

It may be helpful, before your second appointment, to make a note of any questions you think of, however trivial they may seem. It is important to remember to ask the doctor to explain any points that are unclear and to discuss anything you are worried about.

Second appointment

All breast clinics are different and each will have its own way of doing tests and investigations.

If you are asked to attend a second clinic, more X-rays will probably be taken (possibly from different angles) of one or both breasts. A doctor may then examine your breasts for any palpable lump or thickening of the tissue. If the doctor is able to feel anything, you may be given an ultrasound examination (see p. 17), the results of which may be discussed with you at this visit or a subsequent one.

A fine-needle aspiration (see p. 18) may be done to remove a small sample of cells. Occasionally, a core biopsy is done to remove a small piece of tissue from a suspicious lump in the breast (see p. 19). This will probably be at a separate appointment using a local anaesthetic. The cells or tissue sample will have to be examined under a microscope, so another appointment may be made for you to receive the results and discuss them with the doctor. You may be told not to take any aspirin before attending a second breast clinic appointment; this is because aspirin thins the blood, which would cause increased bleeding if a biopsy is done.

A lump that is not palpable (i.e. cannot be felt) may be located using ultrasound or mammography before the biopsy is taken. If the nature of the lump remains unclear following the first investigation, a larger biopsy will be taken. In this case, a fine wire (rather like a very fine crochet hook) is inserted into the suspicious lump, again under ultrasound or mammography guidance. This procedure involves the use of a general anaesthetic while the wire and hook, together with the suspicious area of breast tissue, are removed. X-rays are also usually taken to ensure that the area of suspicious tissue has been removed completely (see 'Stereotactic core biopsy' on p. 19).

Chapter 5

Benign breast disorders

This chapter describes the more common benign causes of pain and swelling in the breast. Although several types of benign tumours of the skin and fatty tissue (lipomas) can occur, these are rare and are therefore not dealt with in detail here.

Breast pain

Breast pain (mastalgia) is a symptom rather than a disease, usually of a minor breast condition, but occasionally of a more serious one. Although most malignant tumours are relatively painless, the presence of breast pain does not necessarily indicate a benign condition.

Breast pain can sometimes be severe and some women who suffer from it cannot bear to be touched or cuddled. It may be cyclical (i.e. related to the menstrual cycle and occurring before or during a period) or non-cyclical, having no obvious menstrual association.

Cyclical breast pain

Cyclical breast pain can often be relieved by taking painkillers such as aspirin, paracetamol, codeine or stronger drugs, prescribed by your doctor. If the breast tissue is inflamed, aspirin will help to deal with this, as it has anti-inflammatory as well as pain-killing properties.

Some women find evening primrose oil an effective treatment for cyclical breast pain and there are some convincing studies that support its use. However, despite some very convincing evidence from placebo-controlled trials, there is still controversy amongst some members of the medical profession about whether the oil itself has any clear medicinal properties. A more expensive form of the active ingredient in evening primrose oil is gamma linoleic acid.

There are several hormonal agents (including contraceptive pills) that can be used to treat very severe period-related breast pain. The sex hormone progesterone can be given in its natural form as Cyclogest pessaries or as one of several synthetic derivatives known as progestogens. Natural or synthetic forms of the hormone oestrogen can also be effective. Other drugs may be prescribed that interfere with the action of the sex hormones produced by the body, for example, in the UK, danazol or bromocriptine, but these can cause fluid retention and headaches and make many women feel generally unwell. They are therefore often given as a last resort for cyclical breast pain that cannot be treated by other means. However, bromocriptine is no longer used in the USA due to some reports there of very serious side-effects. Tamoxifen is also sometimes used to treat cyclical breast pain in the UK, but not in the USA.

Non-cyclical breast pain

If you have non-cyclical breast pain, you will probably be given an examination and mammogram to ensure that there are no signs of breast cancer. Problems such as referred pain from a frozen shoulder, wry neck or twisted back, and infection caused by a virus that attacks the muscles will also have to be ruled out.

This type of breast pain is often more difficult to treat, but in many cases all that is required is reassurance that it is likely to improve with time. When treatment is given, it is the same as that used for cyclical breast pain, although less effective. Good breast support with a well-fitting bra (see p. 6), aspirin and possibly evening primrose oil may help.

There may also be pain with some of the conditions described below, although other symptoms and signs are likely to be apparent.

Breast lumps

Although breast cancer can occur in young women, a lump that develops in a young woman is less likely to be cancerous than one in an older (particularly post-menopausal) woman. However, there are many causes of breast lumps at any age.

Unless a lump can be confirmed as being clearly benign by clinical diagnosis, mammography and fine-needle aspiration (see p. 18) - known as triple assessment - most surgeons will opt to remove it. Some women also prefer to have obviously benign lumps removed and most surgeons will comply with this wish. The operation can normally be performed as minor day-case surgery (see p. 57) under a local or, more usually, a general anaesthetic.

Dysplasia

Dysplasia simply means the abnormal development of tissue. It is a benign condition that becomes apparent as hardening around the edges of the breast, which often occurs in both breasts simultaneously. It is normally associated with age-related changes in the tissue rather than with any serious disease, although it can cause concern to a woman who suddenly discovers it. More localized lumps may be cysts (see p. 31).

Fibroadenosis

Also known as chronic or benign mastitis (a poorly descriptive term that is sometimes used), hyperplastic cystic disease and benign mammary dysplasia, fibroadenosis is a benign condition that usually occurs in women between the ages of 30 and 50. It can also develop around the time of menopause, when it is due to hormone imbalance or to the start of hormone replacement therapy (HRT). Although the cause of fibroadenosis in younger women is unknown, it is possible that it is related to hormone imbalance in this age group as well. This suggestion is based on the facts that its signs and symptoms are related to the menstrual cycle and that it can be induced in men and animals given the female hormone oestrogen. It may be less common in women who have breast-fed their babies.

Symptoms

Fibroadenosis involves 'aberrations in normal development and involution' (known as ANDI). Some parts of the glands of the breast become extensively involuted, whereas in other parts the cells of the ducts increase in both number and size, swell up and block the duct so that the secretions cannot flow or be absorbed and a cyst forms. Alternatively, if there is extensive secretion but the ducts remain open, there may be a discharge from the nipple. Tenderness or lumpiness (or both) is typical.

Fibroadenosis involves the presence of lumps, cysts and irregular breast tissue. Although some degree of lumpiness of the breasts is normal in pre-menopausal women, especially during the last half of each menstrual cycle, one or several persistent lumps appearing before a period and painful, tender breasts could indicate fibroadenosis. Occasionally, there may be an associated clear or brownish discharge from the nipple, and the lymph nodes in the armpits may swell and become tender, although this is more common in duct ectasia (see p. 35).

Diagnosis and treatment

Diagnosis is usually straightforward, but investigations may be necessary to confirm that there is no malignancy. These investigations include fine-needle aspiration biopsy, mammography or ultrasonography (see pp. 14-19). Fibroadenosis is not associated with breast cancer, and surgery to remove part or all of the tissue from a lump should only be necessary if the results of the investigations are inconclusive. A biopsy may also be done for women approaching menopause because their chance of having a cancer is greater.

Although the lumpiness itself requires no special treatment, the breasts should be re-examined by a specialist after 2 or 3 months. This examination should be done during the first half of the menstrual cycle, when there is less normal irregularity of the breast.

If necessary, the symptoms that accompany fibroadenosis, particularly cyclical breast pain, may be relieved by various hormones and 'anti-hormones' such as the drugs danazol and tamoxifen, by evening primrose oil and, possibly, by a low-fat diet (although there is no evidence to substantiate this claim).

Fibroadenosis-like symptoms can also occur in women having HRT, in which case a lower dose of hormone preparation may be required. If pain develops, the HRT may be stopped and then restarted when the pain has cleared.

Cysts

A lump in the breast is most likely to be a fluid-filled cyst or one of a variety of benign tumours that can be treated effectively (see p. 28).

Cysts are most common in women between the ages of 40 and 50, although they may occur at an earlier age in women who have not had children. The majority of cysts are solitary, but some women may have between two and five in one or both breasts.

It is thought that cysts form as an aberration of the normal process of shrinking of the breast that occurs as women get older. Their development appears to be hormone related - possibly associated with the balance between different hormones. Cysts are commonly part of fibroadenosis.

Symptoms

Cysts normally become apparent as smooth lumps in the breast, which may be painful. They are usually quite hard, but can be squeezed between the fingertips. A painless cyst may only be discovered during routine screening by mammography.

Diagnosis and treatment

When a cyst is suspected (and, ideally, when its presence has been confirmed by an ultrasound scan), a needle aspiration (see p. 18) may be performed. The fluid is withdrawn through a needle - the cyst often collapsing like a pricked balloon - and is sent for examination. The remains of the cyst will need to be examined again after about 3 weeks.

Rarely, cancers can form as cysts and for this reason any aspirated bloodstained fluid needs to be examined under a microscope; a biopsy may also be necessary. There is a 10% risk of cancer being associated with a cyst that contains blood, and therefore this type of cyst should be removed. Non-cancerous cysts rarely yield bloody fluid.

Cysts are easily identified on ultrasound or mammography and these investigations may be done when a cyst is suspected in a woman over the age of 35. If the tests reveal a cyst that cannot be felt, a guided needle aspiration may be done (see p. 19).

Although cysts will sometimes refill with fluid after aspiration, further treatment is not normally required. However, a cyst that refills after two or more aspirations may be removed surgically in case it is associated with cancer. Alternatively, a biopsy can be done with a Mammotome® (see p. 19) to remove part of the wall of the cyst, which then collapses. Because of the possible link with cancer, cysts in post-menopausal women (which are uncommon) are often surgically removed.

For women with multiple cysts, drug treatment may help to prevent more developing, although it will not affect those already present.

Fibroadenoma

This is the most common type of benign breast lump, which is usually found in women between the ages of 15 and 25, although it can occur at any age. A fibroadenoma is a fibrous lump of glandular tissue surrounded by a capsule, which can grow to as much as 3-4 cm (1-1.5 inches) across. Fibroadenomas that develop deep within the breast tissue may remain undetected.

Although fibroadenomas are uncommon after menopause, they can occur in women in this age group. It may be that as the breast tissue is replaced by fat, a previously hidden lump is revealed. Some post-menopausal women choose to have a fibroadenoma removed to be absolutely sure of its innocence.

Symptoms

A fibroadenoma may appear as a firm, often hard, painless lump. It is likely to be very mobile and will slip easily out of the fingers when held -

hence the colloquial name 'breast mouse'. In younger women, these tumours rarely grow very large.

Diagnosis and treatment

The results of fine-needle aspiration, mammography or ultrasonography may have to be confirmed by excision biopsy. Surgical removal of fibroadenomas is not usually necessary for medical reasons in younger women, but, as they can be the cause of some anxiety, many women (both young and old) prefer to have them removed. However, very occasionally, a cancer can mimic a fibroadenoma and for this reason it is probably advisable for older women to have any persistent lump removed, particularly if any doubt remains.

Fibroadenomas rarely recur once they have been excised, although others can sometimes form elsewhere in the breast.

Nipple discharge

Some women always have a slight discharge from their nipples and others may develop one during or after pregnancy. Sometimes a profuse, bilateral, bloody discharge occurs during pregnancy. Although nipple discharge is not normally a sign of a serious condition - and is rarely associated with cancer - its cause should always be investigated, particularly if the discharge is blood stained.

Classification

Discharge can occur from one or both nipples, from a single duct or from several, and may or may not contain blood. In some cases, simply avoiding caffeine can lead to a nipple discharge stopping. However, the most common type of discharge is related to mastitis, which is a hormonal condition caused by over-activity in some breast glands, which produce secretions that may be milky, yellow, green or brown. This is commonly associated with discharge from multiple ducts. Discharge from a single duct, particularly if blood stained, is often due to a benign papilloma (see below).

The long-term use of oral contraceptives may be associated with a watery, milky discharge from the nipple, which will cease when the contraceptive is stopped. As the pill is the most effective form of contraceptive, it may be worth putting up with a slight discharge if it does not cause you much distress. However, you should always ask your doctor's advice before stopping any form of contraceptive and make sure you use another suitable type. Paradoxically, a discharge may sometimes also result if the contraceptive pill is stopped.

A milky discharge may occur at puberty and, although it is likely to resolve without the need for treatment, it should be brought to the attention of a doctor.

Very rarely, a profuse, watery, milky discharge may be caused by a pituitary tumour. If a tumour develops in the pituitary gland in the brain, it can cause increased secretion of the hormone prolactin, which triggers the 'let-down' reflex that normally leads to the release of milk during pregnancy.

The following are some other, more important, causes of discharge from the nipple.

Duct papilloma

A papilloma is a benign tumour of any epithelium, which is the layer of cells covering the body's surface and lining most of its hollow structures. In the breast, a papilloma may form in the ducts near the areola. Although it is possible that duct papillomas may be linked to the development of breast cancer in women near menopause, such an association has yet to be proved.

Symptoms

Papillomas occur mostly in women between the ages of 35 and 45. They may cause a bloodstained discharge from the nipple and a lump may be felt on examination.

Diagnosis and treatment

The nipple discharge may be examined under a microscope, but the results are often unreliable. These tumours may show up well on mammography when a radio-opaque substance is injected into the affected duct. This investigation is known as a ductogram and is relatively painless. Ductoscopy, which is similar to a ductogram but involves the use of a very small 'scope' to look inside the duct, is used in some centres in the USA.

Treatment is normally by microdochectomy, which involves expressing the discharge to identify the duct containing the papilloma and then inserting a probe into it. The duct, the inserted probe and the papilloma are then removed.

Duct ectasia and plasma cell mastitis

Duct ectasia is a benign disease in which the ducts just under the nipple become swollen with their own secretions.

Symptoms

The nipple of the affected breast may become inverted and the ducts may secrete a green or yellowish fluid, which can occasionally be bloody. The area around the ducts may become inflamed, giving rise to a type of 'mastitis'.

Plasma cell mastitis can occur if the secretion of duct ectasia leaks out of the ducts and is recognized by the body's defence mechanisms as 'non-self'. The inflammation that results is fought by the plasma cells involved in the reaction against foreign bodies. This can also lead to the formation of abscesses around the areola, particularly if micro-organisms are able to invade the ducts through an inverted nipple. Smoking is a predisposing factor for plasma cell mastitis.

Diagnosis and treatment

Nipple discharge may be the only sign of duct ectasia, but a mammogram is sometimes done to exclude the presence of a cancer and to help confirm the diagnosis.

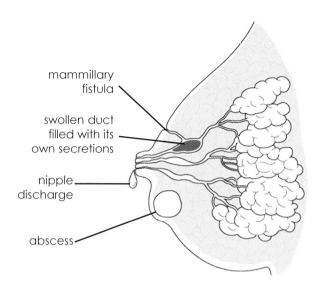

mammillary fistula

swollen duct filled with its own secretions

nipple discharge

abscess

Duct ectasia. *This diagram illustrates some of the complications that can occur in the benign condition of duct ectasia.*

Both duct ectasia and plasma cell mastitis can be difficult to treat, although surgical excision or division of the affected central ducts just under the nipple usually has a good result.

In less serious cases, once reassured that there is no malignant disease present, many women are prepared to put up with the nipple discharge. For those who are not, the major duct complex may be removed surgically and, if necessary, the inverted nipple can be corrected. Loss of or reduction in nipple sensation may sometimes occur following surgery.

If an abscess forms as a result of mastitis, it may need to be surgically incised and drained. It is important for this operation to be performed by an expert surgeon, because simple incision may leave a scar, which continues to drain, causing further nipple discharge. Recurrence of an abscess may result in a mammillary fistula, with intermittent discharge from the areola of the nipple.

Other breast conditions

Eczema

Eczema of the nipple may sometimes occur as a result of irritation caused by the rubbing of clothes (contact eczema) or due to a general skin infection. Some people are born with eczema and it can occur on the nipple, as on any other area of the body.

A specialist can confirm the diagnosis by doing a biopsy of a skin wedge, either under local anaesthetic or, for someone who is particularly anxious or sensitive, as a day-case procedure under a general anaesthetic. Once the cause of the irritation has been removed, a short course of steroid cream may be necessary. Infection can be treated with antibiotics.

Infective 'mastitis'

This can occur in women who are breast-feeding their babies. It may be caused by the transfer of micro-organisms from the hands to the breast through a cracked or inverted nipple, by an infection passed on from the baby's mouth, or by blood-borne infection such as a sore throat.

If the ducts become blocked when a woman is lactating, the milk may stagnate within them and infection can develop. This may cause a dull pain, with inflammation, tenderness, swelling or engorgement of the breast and sometimes an infective discharge from the nipple.

Treatment with antibiotics is usually effective if given early, but breast-feeding will have to stop while the medication is being taken. Breast milk can be expressed with a breast pump, but, as the milk will contain traces of the antibiotic, it should not be given to the baby. Women in this situation should ask their midwives for advice.

Ulcers

On rare occasions, ulcers develop on the nipple during breast-feeding. The baby's sucking can irritate the skin, leading to pain and bleeding from the affected area. Ulcers of this type are more common in fair-skinned women, particularly those with red hair.

Washing and drying the nipple carefully after each feed and the use of Calendula ointment can help to prevent ulcers forming. Once ulcers are present, however, frequent washing with a sterile solution and breast-feeding using an artificial nipple should help. If necessary, breast milk can be expressed with a breast pump.

Abscesses

True breast abscesses are painful and can grow to 5-10 cm (2-4 inches) or more across. They contain pus (which is made up of bacteria and secretions from within the breast) and are distinct from the inflammation due to duct ectasia and plasma cell mastitis. Abscesses can occur anywhere in the breast, the most common cause being blockage and infection of a milk duct during lactation.

Non-lactational abscesses may be associated with plasma cell mastitis and usually occur near the nipple. These are known as subareolar abscesses and are most common in pre-menopausal women. Many are associated with a nipple abnormality such as inversion or retraction.

If treatment is started at an early stage of the development of a lactational abscess, needle aspiration and antibiotics may be sufficient. Otherwise, surgery will be required to incise the abscess and drain away the pus. Expert medical advice should be taken to avoid the risk of mammillary fistulae, which can follow the simple incision of peri-areolar abscesses (see p. 36).

Peripheral breast abscesses can also occur, but these are rare in non-lactating breasts. Early treatment with antibiotics may prevent this type of abscess from forming, but abscesses that do not respond to antibiotics will need to be surgically incised and drained under a general anaesthetic, and in some centres it is common practice to drain all peripheral breast abscesses.

Nipple inversion

If an inverted nipple is stimulated (for example by stroking), it may become everted, but, when the stimulus is removed, the nipple will once again shrink and invert. Permanent inversion can cause difficulties with breast-feeding, but can be corrected by a simple cosmetic operation.

Some women's breasts develop with inverted nipples, but if a previously normal nipple becomes inverted, the cause should be investigated. Although it is likely to be a normal variant, in some cases it may be a sign of an underlying cancer.

Paget's disease

Paget's disease is relatively rare and normally develops in women under the age of 45. It may be confused with eczema, but is a more serious condition and may eventually destroy the nipple completely if left untreated. Most cases of Paget's disease are associated with underlying cancer (see p. 48).

Chapter 6

Breast cancer

A cancer is a collection of cells that are growing and multiplying without proper control. Until recently, when it was overtaken by lung cancer, cancer of the breast was the most common type of cancer affecting women.

Breast cancer is not a single entity; there are various cancers that can develop in the breast, many of which respond well to treatment and may not be life threatening. Early detection and diagnosis are important, as treatment of a small malignant breast tumour at an early stage of development may have a better outcome than for most other types of cancer.

Approximately 75% of breast cancers occur in women over the age of 40; only 2% develop in those younger than 30. Most are in the upper, outer quadrant of the breast. It has been estimated that the average life expectancy of a woman receiving no treatment is about 3 years, although many women live with untreated breast cancer for 10 years or more.

Approximately 1 in 11 women in the UK develop a breast cancer at some time during their lives. Although this figure may seem high, it is less surprising when compared with the figure of 1 in 3 or 4 people developing some form of cancer. However, this statistic needs to be put in context: the most common form of cancer in the UK is cancer of the skin, which in the majority of cases can be treated successfully.

Risk factors

Most of the risk factors associated with the development of breast cancer have been identified by large epidemiological studies, but the actual added risk these factors pose is usually very small, and most women with breast cancer do not have any apparent risk factors. It has also to be borne in mind that women with all the risk factors may not develop breast cancer and those with none of them may do so.

The two biggest risk factors are being a woman and increasing age. Others may include a family history of breast cancer, having children at a late age or not having them at all, and not breast-feeding. The most convincing evidence points towards a genetic predisposition in some women (especially those who develop breast cancer at an early age), some factors in the environment (possibly diet related) and the female hormone oestrogen. Different factors may play a part in different women and some women are more prone than others to developing breast cancer.

Although mammography of young breasts is unreliable, breast screening should ideally begin at the age of 35 for women with substantial risk factors. (In the UK, breast screening currently starts at the age of 50; in the USA, the American Cancer Society recommends it should begin at the age of 40.) Some large centres run special clinics for women in the higher risk categories. It is also very important that women in these categories learn the techniques of breast self-examination and breast awareness (see p. 8).

Although there is controversy about the role of the various possible risk factors, the one thing that does seem clear is that the cause of breast cancer (and of many other cancers) is multifactorial - various different factors combining together in an individual to result in development of the disease. Environmental factors probably act through specific genes in those at risk.

Genetic predisposition

Approximately 5% of breast cancers are related to abnormal genes, notably the *BRAC1* and *BRAC2* genes, particularly in those under the age of 30.

The risk of developing breast cancer is higher in women with a first-order relative (mother or sister) with pre-menopausal breast cancer than in those with an affected relative older than 50. The risk increases for women with two relatives with pre-menopausal breast cancer and in those with the disease in both breasts.

The breast cancer family genes that have been identified are not only found in families with cancer of the breasts, but also in those with ovarian and colon cancer, and women with three or more family members with breast or ovarian cancer have an increased risk of developing breast cancer. Families with these genes should be given specialist advice and counselling at clinics run by geneticists or other qualified professionals.

Geographical differences

Breast cancer is about eight times more common in Northern Europe, North America and Australia than it is in parts of Asia and Africa. However, women who move from low-risk countries (such as Japan) to high-risk countries (such as North America) sometimes show an immediate increase in risk - certainly within one or two generations. Although this does not rule out the possibility of a genetic predisposition, it does seem to indicate an important role for some factor(s) in the environment.

Diet

Some dietary factor(s) may play a part in the increase in risk. Although it is not known how these exert their effects, it may be that they influence hormone synthesis or metabolism. Many foods contain hormones or hormone analogues, either naturally or otherwise. For example, milk is a hormone-derived substance, as, therefore, are butter and cheese etc. Chickens and pigs are often injected with hormones, which may be present in the meat from these animals. The early oral contraceptive pill was made from hormones naturally present in the sweet potato, and ginseng also contains naturally occurring oestrogen. These are just a few examples.

There is evidence to suggest an association between diet and various cancers, including cancer of the breast, although this is not conclusive and some studies have failed to find any such link. Other studies suggest that a diet high in fat and in animal protein (common in most countries in the more affluent West) may be a significant factor in the development of this disease, although there is as yet no conclusive proof of this. Although the

Japanese are now a well-nourished nation, they do not eat a large amount of animal fat and, as mentioned above, do not have a high incidence of breast cancer when living in their own country.

It is also possible (but unproven) that vitamin A may have a protective effect.

The role of female hormones

The fact that breast cancer is about 100 times more common in women than in men suggests a role for the female sex hormones.

Women who had their first period at a young age seem to be more at risk of developing breast cancer, as are those who had their first child late (at 30-34 years old) and those who had a late menopause. Therefore the risk seems to be associated with the number of menstrual cycles a woman has had. Some diets that can lead to obesity, particularly those high in fats, can also lead to an earlier onset of menstruation. Thus, girls in the well-nourished and high socio-economic groups of the industrialized West (where the incidence of breast cancer is high) tend to have their first periods younger than girls in areas of malnutrition (where the disease is less common).

In pre-menopausal women, it is the ovarian oestrogen that is relevant, which is produced for as long as menstruation continues. Breast cancer is less common in women who have had an operation called an oophorectomy to remove their ovaries in their thirties or forties, before their menopause.

In the past, the doses of oestrogen used in hormone replacement therapy (HRT) may have been linked to a slightly increased risk if taken for longer than 10 years. The HRT that is now normally used is a combination of oestrogen and progestogen and the drug doses are much lower. Women who have taken HRT for 10 or more years beyond the expected menopause (at the age of 45-50) have a slow increase in the risk of developing breast cancer, although this is offset by a reduced risk of complications of vascular disease and osteoporosis.

There is considerable controversy surrounding the role of modern contraceptive pills - which also contain a very low hormone dose - but it is possible that they have a slight associated risk when started at an early age and taken for many years. They may, however, reduce the risk for endometrial cancer (cancer of the lining of the womb) and for ovarian cancer. Fibroadenomas in the breast (see p. 32) are also less common in women taking a low-dose contraceptive pill.

Smoking

Cancer cells may spontaneously develop at any time and are usually destroyed by the body's immune system. Smoking suppresses the immune system and therefore it is not surprising that many cancers are more common in those who smoke. However, there is as yet no conclusive evidence to indicate that smoking increases the risk of developing cancer of the breast.

Other risk factors

The strongest risk factor is the previous development of cancer in either the same or the other breast. Other risk factors have been suggested, but with less supporting evidence. For example, there may be a small, but real, link between high alcohol consumption and breast cancer. Stress, either the experience of it or the way it is dealt with, has also been implicated.

Types of breast cancer

Most breast cancers arise from the epithelium of the glandular structure and ducts of the breast; these are known as carcinomas. *Carcinoma in situ* is the term used for a carcinoma that remains in the position in which it developed, with no sign of invasion into the surrounding tissues. *Sarcomas* (tumours arising from the connective tissue) are rare in the breast.

Approximately 90% of breast cancers develop within the epithelial lining of the ducts (ductal carcinomas). Of the remainder, about 5% occur within the lobules of the breast (lobular carcinomas) and these are likely to be associated with second tumours in the same or the other breast. The remaining 5% are a combination of ductal and lobular cancers. There are variant forms of most types of breast cancer, sometimes with a different prognosis from that of the tumours they resemble.

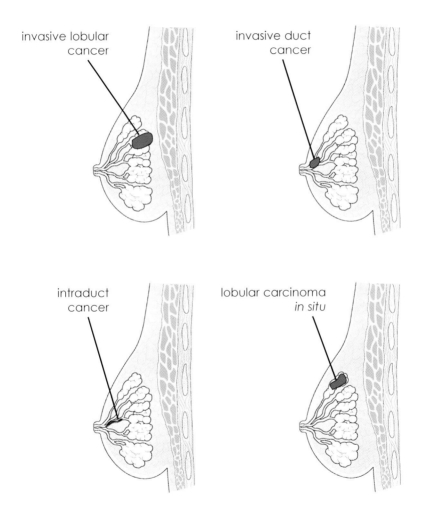

invasive lobular cancer

invasive duct cancer

intraduct cancer

lobular carcinoma *in situ*

Different types of cancer that can occur in the breast.

Different names are used to identify the same cancers in different countries and by different doctors within a country. Confusion is therefore rife - not least amongst the medical profession itself. Where possible, the alternative names are given for the cancers described below.

Breast cancer may be pre-invasive or invasive.

Pre-invasive cancers are either *ductal* or *lobular* carcinomas *in situ*. They are rarely apparent as lumps and are usually detected during breast screening or by chance following biopsy of a benign breast lump.

Invasive cancers can also be either ductal or lobular. Invasive ductal carcinomas account for about 85% of breast cancers, and are classified according to the degree of 'aggressiveness' of their cells, i.e. whether the cells mimic normal tissue closely and whether they tend to adhere to each other:

❖ grade I are well differentiated,

❖ grade II are moderately differentiated,

❖ grade III are undifferentiated (anaplastic) or aggressively spreading.

Invasive lobular carcinomas arise from the lobules of the breast, i.e. more peripherally, and account for about 10% of all breast cancers. They can be multiple and give rise to diagnostic problems because they may not show up on mammography.

Special-type breast cancers

These carry a better prognosis and are classified into *tubular*, *cribriform* or *medullary* cancers, according to the way in which they mimic breast glandular structure. They are often detected on breast screening rather than because they give rise to symptoms.

Other variants

Sometimes a carcinoma may develop within the wall of a cyst, when it is known as an *intracystic* carcinoma. It may be detected when the aspirate of the cyst is heavily blood stained and ultrasound or clinical examination shows that the lump has not disappeared. *Inflammatory* carcinoma is the clinical variant of a very aggressive carcinoma - ductal or lobular - which causes the breast to become swollen, red and warm, and sometimes the skin shows oedema, like the skin of an orange - known as *peau d'orange* (see p. 8). This type of cancer usually requires pre-treatment before surgery.

Ductal tumours

These usually develop as a hard, painless swelling in women near or past their menopause. They often occur in the upper, outer quadrant of the breast and may spread into the surrounding fat. There may also be malignant cells in the nearby lymph vessels and blood capillaries.

There is a very slow-growing tumour that may cause contraction and deformity of the breast in elderly women. It is often only found on mammography and can remain localized in the breast for many years. This type of tumour was previously known as an atrophic *scirrhous* carcinoma.

Medullary carcinoma
Also called *lymphocytic* or *encephaloid* carcinoma, this is softer and more rapidly growing than the scirrhous tumour. It usually has a better prognosis than scirrhous carcinoma, because of the body's immune reaction to it.

Inflammatory carcinoma/carcinoma of pregnancy and lactation
These tumours may resemble breast abscesses. They grow rapidly and may cause the breast to become hot and tender. They do not normally become apparent until a late stage. Chemotherapy and radiotherapy are often given before surgery to 'down-stage' the tumour.

Papillary carcinoma

Papillary carcinomas are a rare variant of the special-type carcinomas, with a good prognosis. They develop as a mass of cells within the lumen of a duct and present early with a bloody nipple discharge. They are much less common than the benign duct papillomas (see p. 34).

Cystic carcinoma

Cystic carcinomas are rare (only about 1% of all breast cancers), but they have a variable prognosis. When aspirated, the fluid they contain is bloody and can be seen under a microscope to contain malignant cells.

Lobular tumours

Cancers in the lobules of the breast are 10-20 times less common than ductal carcinomas. The prognoses are similar, but lobular carcinomas are more likely to occur in both breasts, sometimes several being present at the same time.

Paget's disease of the nipple

Paget's disease is a pre-cancerous condition that normally occurs in women over the age of 45. It is caused by the growth of a ductal cancer onto the areola. It is quite a rare condition, which may be confused with eczema, but which spreads over the areolar region far less quickly and may destroy the nipple completely over a long period of time. If left untreated, it never heals and eventually forms an ulcer. Typically, only one breast is affected, with a persistent, scaly rash on the nipple or a weeping eczema, often with destruction or distortion of the nipple itself.

Wedge excision of the affected area or the examination of scraped cells under a microscope will confirm the diagnosis. This is a far more serious disease than eczema, and treatment may involve complete removal of the affected breast. Persistent redness or nipple discharge should always be reported to a doctor, even if you have eczema elsewhere on your body, as the cancer associated with Paget's disease is not necessarily palpable.

How breast cancer spreads

Cells from the primary tumour can spread to other parts of the body to produce secondary tumours. The process is known as metastasis and the secondary tumours are called metastases. Metastasis can occur in the following ways.

❖ By *direct extension*: the cancer grows into the surrounding breast tissue.

❖ By *lymphatic spread*: this is either due to permeation or to clumps of cells breaking off and travelling in the lymph down the lymphatic vessels to the lymph glands. Although the lymph glands act as a filter, the cancer cells may take over, invade and colonize the glands.

❖ Into *blood vessels*: cancer cells may be deposited in the bone marrow, bones, lungs and liver.

❖ By *spread across body cavities*: for example across the membrane that covers the lungs (the pleura).

The most common sites of metastases in breast cancer are bone, lung and liver and, less commonly, the brain. However, the lymph nodes are affected first, malignant cells becoming lodged in them and multiplying to form further tumours.

Although both breasts can be affected simultaneously, it is more usual for the second breast to become involved after a period of years, if at all. Rarely, spread to the second breast occurs via the lymph vessels.

Differentiation of carcinomas

The differentiation of a carcinoma depends on the nature of its cells. A pathologist will examine the cells of a malignant tumour and report on their size and regularity, the condition of the nucleus and the amount of nuclear material, and on whether the cells adhere to each other. On the basis of these factors, malignant tumours are classified as:

❖ well differentiated: containing easily identifiable cells that clearly resemble the tissue from which they were derived (grade I);

❖ moderately differentiated: an intermediate form (grade II);

❖ undifferentiated: containing a mixture of cells whose tissue of origin is difficult to identify (grade III).

The prognosis for a well-differentiated cancer is always better than that for a poorly differentiated one. This grading of carcinomas is important for treatment as well as for prognosis.

Staging

Cancers are staged to measure how far they have progressed. An early-stage breast cancer is one that is confined to the breast; an advanced-stage cancer has spread to other parts of the body. There are several different systems for staging breast cancers, some of which are more complicated than others. Staging is used to help decide on the most appropriate treatment as well as allowing an assessment to be made of the likely outcome of that treatment. The treatment given for a breast cancer at an early stage is often different from that required for more advanced disease.

There are various methods of assessing the outcome for a woman with breast cancer, based on factors such as:

❖ whether she is pre-menopausal or post-menopausal (her hormone status);

❖ the size of the tumour and whether it has invaded the lymphatic or blood vessels;

❖ the differentiation of the tumour (see above);

❖ whether the tumour has spread to the axillary lymph nodes;

❖ whether the tumour is confined to the ducts of the breast (intraductal cancer).

The last factor is important because complete cure is usually possible for tumours that have not spread beyond a duct, by surgically removing the tissue containing the duct and the growth within it. Intraductal tumours, once removed, do not tend to recur.

Staging depends on the size and fixity of the cancer and on whether or not the lymph nodes are involved. The TNM (tumour-nodes-metastases) staging system classifies cancers in the following way, tumours at stage 1 (confined to the breast) having the best prognosis.

Tumour

T0   No palpable tumour
T1   Tumour size 2 cm; no fixation
T2   Tumour size more than 2 cm/less than 5 cm; no fixation
T3   Tumour size more than 5 cm
T4   Tumour of any size; fixation to the chest wall or ulceration of the skin

Lymph nodes

N0   No palpable axillary nodes
N1a Palpable nodes that do not appear to contain tumour
N1b Palpable nodes that are thought to contain tumour
N2   Node size more than 2 cm or fixed to one another or to deep structures
N3   Supraclavicular or infraclavicular nodes

Metastases

M0   No apparent distant metastases
M1   Distant metastases

Prognosis

The prognosis for a particular breast cancer depends on its cellular type, stage and differentiation. Of particular importance is the extent of the tumour, in terms of lymph node involvement, its size and degree of differentiation. The prognosis is important not only in determining the outlook for the woman, but also in determining the type of treatment required.

Treatment

This section gives only a brief overview of the treatments for breast cancer; more detailed discussion of the treatments available for benign and malignant breast lumps can be found in Chapters 9 and 12.

There have always been conflicting views amongst members of the medical profession about how to treat breast cancer. Some specialists believe that radical treatment is best, others that a combination of less surgically aggressive treatments is as effective, and others that treatment has no effect on the course of the disease in some forms of cancer. To try to deal with this problem, trials were set up some years ago in the UK and in many other countries in which women with breast cancer took part, having given their informed consent. The surgeons involved in these trials could no longer choose a treatment regimen for their breast cancer patients, but had to follow a predetermined plan, based on statistical data, which provided a particular type of treatment for a particular type of cancer. On the basis of the results of these trials, national guidelines have now been established in the UK for breast cancer treatment.

There are several different operations for treating breast cancer, which are described in detail in Chapter 9. The decision to operate will depend on the stage at which the tumour is first detected and on which parts of the body are involved.

The two main types of treatment for breast cancer are:

❖ *surgery*, which involves removal of the tumour as well as of some or all of the lymph nodes in the armpit so that the disease can be staged, and

❖ *adjuvant therapy*, which includes endocrine or hormone treatment, radiotherapy and chemotherapy.

You can, of course, choose to have no treatment, although without it the tumour may eventually erupt through the skin, forming ulcers on the breast, and metastases may develop.

Surgery

The operation performed for a palpable lump will be one of the following:

❖ *breast conservation*, involving a wide local excision to remove the lump and an area of the surrounding tissue;

❖ *simple mastectomy*, involving removal of all the breast tissue including the nipple.

The decision about which operation is most appropriate will be based on consideration of the pathology and size of the tumour, its site, the likely cosmetic result following conservation, whether there are multiple tumours in the breast, and your own wishes.

If you have a non-palpable lump - for example if you have no apparent clinical abnormality but were found to have an abnormality on screening that was subsequently proven to be malignant - you will go first to the radiology department, where the tumour will be marked by the insertion of a very fine wire (like a fuse wire) under a local anaesthetic. Your operation will then take place under a general anaesthetic later the same day.

During surgery, the surgeon will try to remove at least four lymph nodes or will excise a block of the axillary fat containing all of them, in order to obtain a sample of the lymph nodes for assessment. Sometimes, the axillary lymph nodes are removed during a second operation if a definite diagnosis cannot be made. If breast conservation surgery has been carried out and, after pathological examination, the surgeon feels that an inadequate margin of tissue was removed from around the tumour, a further wide excision of breast tissue may be done subsequently.

Breast conservation: wide local excision of the breast and axillary node sampling

This operation involves the removal of the lump itself rather than of the entire breast. It may be the treatment of choice for single tumours up to about 2 cm (about ¾ inch) in diameter. Surgery is followed by radiotherapy, which is particularly important if the lymph nodes are involved. Women who have had this operation require long-term follow-up.

The cosmetic appearance is usually good and the scar is small. However, if several axillary lymph nodes have been removed, there may be subsequent swelling of the arm and hand (known as lymphoedema, see p. 96), because the lymph can no longer drain rapidly from the area.

Simple mastectomy

In simple or total mastectomy, the entire breast is removed, usually with some or all of the axillary lymph nodes. Breast reconstruction is often possible following this operation. The risk of lymphoedema in the arm is increased if all the axillary lymph nodes are removed or if some of them are excised for staging and then radiotherapy is given. Radical mastectomy (which involves the removal of the breast and both pectoral muscles) is now very rarely done, and the Patey or modified radical mastectomy (which involves the removal of the breast and only the smaller pectoral muscle) is also uncommon.

Adjuvant treatment

An adjuvant treatment is one that is given in combination with another type of treatment - in this case surgery - to maximize its benefits.

Hormone therapy

It is now common to assess the sensitivity of breast cancers to see whether there are receptors for the hormones oestrogen and progesterone on the outside of the cells. If the tumour is positive (sensitive), hormone therapy can be given. Hormone therapy alters the body's levels of the naturally occurring female hormones or prevents them being taken up by cancer cells.

The main drug used for hormone therapy is tamoxifen, which is antagonistic to oestrogen and blocks the receptors for it. Alternatives are goserelin (Zoladex), which induces a temporary menopause, and the pituitary hormones megestrol (Megace - a synthetic form of progesterone) and anastrozole (Arimidex - one of a group of medications that inhibit the enzyme aromatase, which is important in the synthesis of these hormones). If the cancer recurs after treatment with one drug, a different one may then be used. (Hormone therapy is discussed in more detail in Chapter 12.)

Radiotherapy

Radiotherapy is used as an adjuvant to breast conservation surgery for invasive breast cancer, and sometimes after mastectomy for a tumour that was very close to the pectoral muscles of the chest wall. Although it may be used when malignant cells have spread to the lymph nodes in the axilla and above the clavicle, this is not routine practice.

Radiotherapy can also help to alleviate the pain of extensive breast cancer that cannot be cured, particularly where there is localized spread of the cancer to the bones, such as in the spine. It may be the treatment of choice for women who are unfit for surgery and for those in whom secondary tumours have developed in the bones and skin (see also p. 104). The X-ray beam can be directed onto the tumour itself, making it shrink and helping to relieve the pain it was causing. If a breast tumour shrinks enough, a mastectomy may be feasible at a later date.

Radiotherapy is given externally or, less commonly, via an internal implant of radioactive material. (A more detailed discussion of radiotherapy can be found in Chapter 12.)

Chemotherapy

Chemotherapy is drug treatment using a combination of anti-cancer (cytotoxic) drugs that destroy cancer cells. It may be used as:

❖ *neoadjuvant treatment*, given before surgery to downgrade the stage of the tumour, or as

❖ *adjuvant treatment*, given when the tumour is extensive and there is lymph node involvement, particularly in a younger, pre-menopausal woman and for cancers that are oestrogen insensitive. It is given after surgery, either alone or in conjunction with radiotherapy.

One of the most commonly used combinations of cytotoxic drugs is CMF - cyclophosphamide, methotrexate and fluorouracil. Alternatives include FEC - fluorouracil, epirubicin and cisplatin - and the newer chemotherapy agents such as paclitaxel (Taxol) and docetaxel (Taxotere). (Further details of chemotherapy are given in Chapter 12.)

Choosing a treatment

All women should have a say in what form of treatment - if any - they receive and an opportunity to discuss their options with their family before making a decision. It is important that you are aware of all the options available to you and that you take account of any advice your specialist has given you.

The results of clinical trials indicate that the rates of survival and of local recurrence of breast cancer are similar whether treatment is by mastectomy or wide local excision. In some cases, however, depending on the site, size and spread of the cancer, mastectomy is recommended.

It is usually possible - and important - for women with suspected or proven breast cancer and their families to receive counselling, and many hospitals now have specially trained breast care nurses who can provide valuable support and information (see p. 21).

Chapter 7

Going in to hospital for an operation

Whatever type of breast surgery you are having, you will probably be admitted to hospital as soon as possible after your clinic visit. In almost all cases, the speed with which your hospital admission is arranged will reflect an understanding of the stress involved for you and your family, rather than any urgent need for your operation to be done immediately.

You should get a letter from the hospital telling you the date of your operation and any other details you need to know. Many hospitals also send out leaflets explaining their admission procedures and giving advice on what to take in with you. The hospital's breast care or other specialist nurse will also send you any specific information that may be useful.

Length of stay

Your length of stay in hospital will depend on the type of operation you are having. For an operation to remove a small breast lump, day-case surgery may be appropriate (see below), or you may stay in hospital overnight afterwards. If you are having a wide local excision to remove a breast lump and some axillary lymph nodes, you may have to stay in hospital for a couple of days. However, most operations in the UK are increasingly being done as day-case surgery or with a single night in hospital, whenever possible. A more extensive mastectomy operation may involve at least 3-4 days in hospital or, at some hospitals, up to 8 days.

During your operation, one or two small tubes may be inserted into your wound to drain any blood or fluid that collects after the tissues have been cut and that cannot escape once the wound has been sewn. You will not be able to leave hospital until drainage stops and the tubes can be removed, which may take anything from 1 to 7 days.

Day-case surgery

If you are having day-case surgery for a non-palpable lump, you will go to the radiology department in the morning so that the lump can be located and a fine wire will be inserted (see p. 26). You will then have your operation under a general anaesthetic in the afternoon.

To be suitable for day-case surgery, you must be physically fit and mentally prepared and must have suitable transport to get home and an adult to stay with you for at least the first night. Women with co-existent disease (such as heart or lung disease) cannot be considered for day-case surgery, as they require full assessment and in-patient treatment.

The majority of women are able to go home after day-case surgery, but if you are unwell after the anaesthetic, are vomiting or have a wound problem, you will need to stay in hospital overnight. Even after more extensive operations, day-case surgery is often suitable, and it is sometimes possible to go home with drains in place, which can be managed by a district nurse.

What to take into hospital

The information in this section applies if you are due to stay in hospital for at least one night. There are very few things you will need.

❖ *Nightclothes.* Loose, comfortable nightclothes are best. You will be given a hospital gown to wear during the operation itself.

❖ *Slippers.*

❖ *Dressing gown.*

❖ *Towel and washing things.*

❖ *Money.* A small amount of money may be useful for newspapers and the telephone. Large sums of money, wallets and handbags should not be taken into hospital, as these may have to be kept in an unlocked cabinet by your bed. If you do have to take any valuables or large sums of money into hospital, you should give them to the nurse in charge of your ward when you are admitted. You will be given a receipt listing each item, which you should keep safe so that you can collect your possessions when you are discharged. However, hospital authorities strongly discourage people from bringing anything of great value with them unless absolutely necessary.

Jewellery

Whenever possible, all jewellery should be left at home. Although wedding rings may be worn during an operation, there is a risk that any jewellery you take off before surgery may be lost or stolen. If you have to take any jewellery into hospital, it should be given to the ward sister for safe keeping.

Wedding rings, or any other rings that are very precious to you or that cannot be removed, will be covered with adhesive tape before your operation, because metal can cause electrical burns or electric shocks during the process of electrocautery that is used to control bleeding during surgery. (Electrocautery involves the use of an electric current to heat the tip of the instrument that shrivels and seals the little blood vessels and stops them bleeding.)

❖ *Books, magazines, puzzles, knitting.* There will inevitably be periods of waiting between visits from medical staff before your operation and you may want something to occupy you during this time.

❖ *Clothes to wear to go home.* Following a mastectomy, you should be fitted with a soft, temporary prosthesis before you go home. The breast care nurse or ward sister will fit this inside your bra as an interim measure until you are given a permanent prosthesis - about 6-8 weeks after the operation, when the wound has completely healed. Therefore, if you are having a mastectomy, you should take into hospital with you a well-fitting, comfortable bra that is not wired or low cut, preferably made of Lycra or elastic to provide support, and in good condition. You may also be asked to take a tight-fitting T-shirt or similar garment to wear while the nurse is matching the shape of the prosthesis to that of your other breast, although you will probably be more comfortable wearing a loose shirt or sweater to go home in.

❖ *Drugs you are already taking.* Once your admission has been arranged, your family doctor will have been asked to fill in a form stating all the drugs you are taking and their doses. You may also be asked to take your drugs with you when you go into hospital so that their dosages can be checked and so that you can continue to be given any that you need to keep taking. All your drugs will be kept for you during your stay, because you must only take those that are given to you by medical staff. If you are asked to take your own drugs into hospital, these should be returned to you before you leave.

❖ *Admission letter.* An admission letter will have been sent to you from the hospital and you should take this with you when you are admitted for your operation.

Hospital staff

The ward of a hospital is a busy place and can seem confusing and frightening. It may help to have an idea of the different medical staff you are likely to meet.

❖ *The breast care nurse.* Almost all hospitals have designated breast care nurses and their numbers are increasing as the contribution they can make to the care of women with breast cancer is recognized. Breast care nurses are experienced nurses who have chosen to specialize in caring for women with breast cancer and breast diseases. They are able to provide support, information and advice about the diseases themselves as well as about practical issues. Many women find it easier to talk to their breast care nurse than to their consultant and feel less embarrassed about asking questions and for explanations of things they have not understood. A breast care nurse will also be available to talk to your relatives; many arrange appointments for women and their partners so that they can talk to them both together and separately.

It is not necessary to make an appointment through your family doctor to see your breast care nurse. Apart from visiting women every day during their stay in hospital, breast care nurses can also arrange home visits for those women who want them.

❖ *Nurses*. The uniforms worn to distinguish nurses of different ranks vary from hospital to hospital, but all nurses wear badges, which state clearly their name and sometimes their grade. There are, of course, both male and female nurses, although women are still in the majority.

The ward may also have several *nursing auxiliaries*. These are not trained nurses, but deal with any non-medical jobs and help with the basic care of patients.

❖ *Doctors*. Each consultant surgeon in a hospital heads a team of doctors of different ranks, sometimes known as a 'firm'. You may meet some or all of them. These doctors can, of course, be men or women.

❖ *Anaesthetists*. Anaesthetists are highly trained doctors who specialize in giving anaesthetics and in pain relief. An anaesthetist will visit you before your operation to discuss any relevant details, such as any anaesthetics you have had in the past and any drugs you may be taking (see p. 65).

❖ *Medical social workers*. If any problems arise at home during your stay in hospital, or if you are concerned about being able to manage on your own once you return home, you can ask to talk to a medical social worker. Medical social workers work in close partnership with other medical staff in the hospital and will be able to give you advice and practical support.

If necessary, nursing staff may be able to organize 'meals on wheels' or a home help for you if you will be in hospital for only a short time. They can also arrange for a social worker to visit you at home if required.

Before the operation

Admission to the ward

When you arrive at the hospital, you should report to the main reception desk with your admission letter. The staff there will check your details and tell you which ward to go to. Once on the ward, the ward clerk will deal with the clerical side of your admission, filling in the necessary forms with you. You will then be allocated a bed and introduced to a nurse who will admit you to the ward, look after you during your stay and co-ordinate your discharge when the time comes. You will be allocated another nurse for other working shifts.

You will be asked to help your nurse draw up a care plan when you are admitted to the ward, and should include in it details of any preferences or dislikes you have, for example if you prefer to sleep with several pillows, if there are certain foods you do not want, or if you have any ailments other than that for which you are having surgery, such as arthritis. Your care plan may be kept at the bottom of your bed, but, wherever it is, it is available for you to read. Nursing staff may tick off a checklist as they carry out the various procedures and will update the care plan with you as the need arises. Do tell the nurse if you have any problems or if you are anxious about any aspect of your hospital stay.

As you are admitted to the ward, the nurse will take notes of your personal details and explain the ward procedures to you. Your discharge will also be planned at this time. The nursing staff will need to be sure that someone will be able to collect you and take you home when the time comes. If this is not possible, hospital transport may be arranged for you. Also, if you are due to go home the day after your operation, your nurse will want to be sure you can manage. The effects of anaesthetic gases, and of other agents used by the anaesthetist, can remain for several days and, although you may feel you are fully recovered, your reaction times will be slow and you may continue to feel sick and light-headed for at least the next couple of days. If you are elderly, it is particularly important to have someone to help you for a day or two after your operation. All this will be taken into account as you and the nurse plan your discharge.

The nurse will measure your blood pressure, temperature and pulse. A sample of your urine may be taken for analysis to make sure you do not have diabetes or any disorder of the kidneys that would complicate the operation. You may also be weighed, because the anaesthetist may need to know your weight in order to be able to calculate the appropriate dose of anaesthetic for you.

You will be shown to your bed on the ward and told of any ward details, such as meal times and where to find the toilets, day room etc.

Anti-embolism stockings

Once you are settled on the ward, a nurse will probably measure your legs for the stockings you will be given to wear during your operation. These Thrombo-Embolic Deterrent Stockings (TEDS) used to be worn only by patients having major operations to help prevent blood clots forming in the veins deep within their legs as they lay motionless on the operating table, sometimes for several hours. However, they are now used routinely as a precaution in almost all operations, even those that last for less than an hour. Although the stockings may feel uncomfortable, there is no doubt as to their value.

The nurse will measure your calf, thigh and the length of your leg and will give you a pair of stockings of the correct size. Although you will probably be given the stockings on admission to the ward, you may not need to put them on until you are preparing to go to the operating room. You should keep them on until you are up and about again after your operation.

The normal activity of the muscles in the legs helps to keep the blood moving through them. During long periods of bed rest or anaesthesia, these muscles are inactive and the circulation of blood in the legs slows down. A blood clot is thus more likely to form, which can block the passage of blood through the vein. This is known as a thrombosis. If pieces of this clot break off, they form emboli. Even one embolus may have serious consequences if it travels through the circulation and lodges in a vital organ such as the lung. Anti-embolism stockings improve the return of venous blood to the heart and thus help to prevent blood clots forming.

Heparin injections

High-risk patients, such as those with a previous history of deep vein thrombosis (DVT), may be given subcutaneous injections of a low dose of low molecular weight heparin during their hospital stay. Heparin is an anticoagulant, found naturally within the body, which thins the blood and helps to prevent blood clots forming.

Heparin injections are usually started with the pre-medication ('pre-med.') and are given once a day until patients are mobile again after surgery. Although a very fine needle is used (which is inserted into the fat, usually in the thigh), small bruises can develop around the injection site.

Ward visits

A *doctor* will visit you on the ward before your operation to take details of your medical history, including any allergies you may have and any drugs you are taking, and to examine you. Your family doctor may have already filled in a form giving the names and dosages of any drugs you have been prescribed and you should have been told what to do about these. Do not forget to tell the hospital doctor of any other drugs you have been taking that your family doctor may not know about, such as vitamin supplements, cough medicines, aspirins etc., which are available from the chemist without the need for prescription.

If you normally take a contraceptive pill or tablets for hormone replacement therapy (HRT), you may have been told to stop these for a time before your operation. If you are still taking them when you enter hospital, for example if you have been called for your operation at short notice, you should tell the doctor. Contraceptive pills used to contain much larger amounts of hormones than are present in the more modern ones, and these were sometimes associated with complications from blood clots. The newer pills are almost entirely free from these risks, but some surgeons still prefer their patients to stop taking them for at least a month before surgery, if possible.

A medical examination will also be done to identify any illness or infection you may have that could complicate the use of a general anaesthetic. If you are over 50 years of age or a heavy smoker, you will probably have to have a chest X-ray and an electrocardiogram (ECG) so that any potential anaesthetic complications due to breathing or heart problems can be picked up.

If you are having a palpable lump removed from your breast, the doctor will try to locate it and will mark the appropriate area on the surface of your breast with an indelible felt-tip pen. If the entire breast is to be removed, the appropriate one will be identified in the same way.

The *surgeon* who is to perform your operation may also visit you on the ward to check that all is well, and the *anaesthetist* will probably come to see you to ask about anything that may be relevant to the choice of anaesthetic given to you.

Anaesthetics have improved considerably during the last few years and a 'pre-med.' is now not always given routinely. If you are very anxious and need something to relax you, you may be given some form of sedative, by mouth or injection, 2 or 3 hours before the operation. If you enter hospital the day before your operation and think that you will be too anxious to sleep that night, you can ask the house surgeon or senior house officer for something to help you.

A *breast care nurse* will visit you on the ward before and after your operation as often as is necessary. She will be able to answer any questions you may have and will be happy to talk to members of your family. Do discuss with her anything that is worrying you; she will be very experienced and will be able to explain things clearly and simply.

Consent forms

The surgeon who is to perform your operation will ask you to sign a consent form. Although it can be assumed that your consent to the operation is implied by the fact that you have entered hospital willingly, consent forms are widely used. Before signing this form, your operation must have been explained to you and you must understand fully what it entails. You may need to have several discussions with the specialist and nurse counsellor before you have a clear idea of what is involved in your operation. The operating details must be written in full and the breast that is to be operated on must be clearly identified. You are also giving your permission for the doctors to take whatever action they feel to be appropriate should some emergency arise during your operation and for any necessary anaesthetic to be given to you. Do read this form carefully and ask the doctor to explain anything you do not understand.

'Nil by mouth'

This is a term that means that neither food nor drink must be swallowed. To prevent you vomiting and the risk of choking on your vomit while you are anaesthetized, you will be told not to eat or drink anything for 4-6 hours before your operation. You will, however, be able to have a few sips of water with any tablets you need to take, such as those for blood pressure etc. If you are admitted the night before surgery, you will be able to have supper on the ward. If you enter hospital in the morning and your operation is to be that afternoon, you should not eat or drink for about 6 hours beforehand.

Shaving

Many women will already have shaved their armpits before coming in to hospital. If you have not done so, you will probably be given either a disposable razor or clippers to shave the hair from the entire armpit area. Although hair clippers are preferable, because they prevent the skin being 'nicked' by leaving a layer of short hair on it, thus reducing the risk of post-operative infection, they are quite expensive. Disposable razors are therefore more commonly used. Occasionally, women are given a hair-removing (depilatory) cream.

Apart from allowing the surgeon a clear view of the area of operation, shaving also makes the removal of any adhesive wound dressing less painful.

If you are anxious about doing the shaving yourself, do ask a nurse if someone can do it for you. Arthritis of the hands, for example, can make this a difficult task.

Smoking

If you are a heavy smoker, you will be advised not to smoke in the hours before your operation. (It is, of course, much better to stop smoking some months before any type of surgery.) The carbon monoxide contained in cigarette smoke poisons the blood by replacing some of the oxygen that is carried in it, which is vital to processes such as wound healing.

Waiting

It may seem that you have been admitted to hospital unnecessarily early and you may find you have to wait on the ward with little to do. Apart from having to be seen by all the medical staff mentioned above, who are responsible for many other patients as well, time will also have been allowed for the assessment of any medical problems you may have and for the results of any blood tests to be received.

Sometimes operations have to be cancelled at the last moment if an emergency has arisen and an earlier operation has taken longer than expected. Your operation may have to be postponed, perhaps for a few hours or until the following day, but hospital staff understand the stress that is caused by a cancelled operation and it is extremely unlikely that you would be sent home.

You will probably be given only an approximate time for your operation, being told if it is scheduled for the morning or afternoon. Surgery being done before yours may take longer than expected if complications arise.

Leaving the ward for your operation

Before being taken from the ward to the anaesthetic room or operating theatre, you will be given a hospital gown to wear and will be asked to put on your anti-embolism stockings. A plastic-covered bracelet bearing your name and an identifying hospital number will be attached to one or both of your wrists. You will then be taken from the ward on a hospital trolley.

Chapter 8

Anaesthesia

An anaesthetist will probably visit you on the ward before your operation. Anaesthetists are hospital doctors who have been trained in the special skills of giving drugs that cause loss of sensation or consciousness, or both (anaesthetics), and those that block feelings of pain (analgesics). Anaesthesia is a vital part of any operation and a great deal of time and trouble will be taken to make sure you receive the anaesthetic that best suits you.

The pre-anaesthetic visit

The main reason for the anaesthetist's visit before your operation is to decide what type of anaesthesia would be safest for you. This visit also gives you the opportunity to discuss any problems or worries you may have concerning your anaesthesia.

The anaesthetist will ask you several questions about any anaesthetics you have had before, any drugs you are taking, and about your general health. It is important that you answer these questions as fully as possible. You should also mention to the anaesthetist if you have any false or crowned teeth. False teeth and dental bridges have to be removed before you go into the operating theatre because a broken or loose tooth can be inhaled into the lungs during surgery.

If you have had any problems in the past such as an allergy to a particular anaesthetic, it will be helpful if you know the name of the drug concerned or the hospital where the operation was carried out. The appropriate records can then be checked to make sure another type of anaesthetic is used for your breast operation. You should also tell the anaesthetist if you know of any other member of your family who has reacted against a particular drug, as you may have the same problem.

The anaesthetist may also want to examine you and to look at the results of any tests you have had. There are different types of anaesthetic that can be used for breast operations (see below), and some health problems will preclude the use of certain ones.

General anaesthesia

Virtually all breast operations require a general anaesthetic; the only exception may be for a biopsy, which can be performed in an out-patient department using a local anaesthetic. A general anaesthetic will put you to sleep and abolish any feeling in your body. It can be given in two different ways.

❖ *Intravenous* anaesthetics can be injected into a vein via a plastic tube inserted into your hand or arm, and will put you to sleep within a few seconds.

❖ *Inhalational* anaesthetics are gases that you breathe in through a facemask and that act within 1-2 minutes. As the use of a facemask can cause some people to panic, it is not normally applied until you are asleep.

During the operation, the anaesthetist will make sure you stay asleep by giving you more drugs as necessary.

Risks of general anaesthesia

People with certain medical conditions, such as heart or lung disease, may not be given general anaesthetics, as they are potentially at greater risk.

Some people are afraid of being put to sleep by a general anaesthetic because they fear the possibility of never waking up or of suffering brain damage. General anaesthetics are very much safer today than they were even 20 years ago, because of the many advances in techniques and drugs. Therefore, their risks are small, although they do have to be borne in mind (see p.100). If you are worried about this, you should discuss with your anaesthetist the possibility of an alternative.

Local anaesthesia

When the general anaesthetic has taken effect and you are asleep, the anaesthetist or surgeon may inject some local anaesthetic into the area to be operated on. This is the same type of drug that a dentist uses to numb the teeth before a filling. The injection will provide you with pain relief after the operation, for about 4-6 hours.

Other medication

In some hospitals, a pre-medication drug ('pre-med.') is given routinely to patients to reduce their anxiety before an operation. A 'pre-med.' is given by mouth, as tablets or syrup, or by injection several hours before the operation. It will probably make you feel sleepy and relaxed.

You may be asked whether you would like to have a 'pre-med.' or you may have to ask for one yourself if you feel anxious and have not been offered one. You can, of course, also say that you do not want one if they are given routinely in your hospital. The anaesthetist will be able to discuss this with you.

You may also be given any drugs that you normally take, such as diuretics ('water tablets') or medication to reduce high blood pressure.

Before your operation

You will be told not to have anything to eat or drink for at least 6 hours before your operation ('nil by mouth', see p. 66). The reason for this is that any food or drink left in your stomach when you are anaesthetized could cause you to be sick.

While you are still on the ward, you will be given your 'pre-med.', if you are having one, and any medicines you normally take. You will then be taken to the operating theatre, probably on a hospital trolley. You may go first into the anaesthetic room or straight into the operating theatre to be given your anaesthetic.

The anaesthetist, or an assistant, will ask you several questions to confirm your identity and make sure that you are the right person in the right place. Your identity bands will also be checked. Many people have many types of operations each day in a hospital, and these checks, which may be repeated, are essential to make sure no mistakes are made.

The anaesthetist will then fit various monitoring devices to watch over you while you are asleep. A probe (a pulse oximeter) may be attached to your finger to measure the amount of oxygen in your blood; some sticky pads may be put on your chest so that your heartbeat can be recorded on an electrocardiograph; and a cuff may be put around your arm to measure your blood pressure. All these monitoring devices enable the anaesthetist to make sure that the anaesthetic remains effective and that you remain well during surgery.

A plastic cannula will be put into a vein in the back of your hand, and any drugs will be introduced into your body through this.

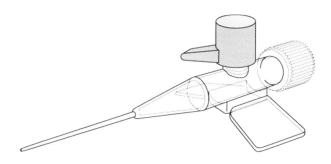

A butterfly cannula. *Drugs are introduced into the body through the cannula during an operation. This is an example of a typical cannula, which is inserted into a vein, usually in the back of the hand.*

Once the anaesthetist is happy with the readings from the monitors, your anaesthesia can start.

Anaesthesia

The anaesthetist will remain with you throughout your operation to make sure you are asleep and that the function of your heart and lungs is satisfactory. Once the anaesthetic has been injected into the tube in your hand or arm, you will fall asleep within seconds. The drug that makes you go to sleep may sting a little as it enters the vein from the cannula, but this feeling does not last long.

Several different types of drugs will be given to you during your operation:

❖ *induction* agents to bring on sleep,

❖ *maintenance* agents to keep you asleep,

❖ *analgesics* to stop you feeling pain after the operation,

❖ *anti-emetics* to help stop you feeling sick after the operation.

If local anaesthetic is injected into the wound during surgery, you will have little or no pain when you wake up.

After your operation

When your operation is over, the anaesthetist will stop giving you the drugs that were keeping you asleep, and you will probably be taken to a recovery room. The nurses in the recovery room are specially trained to care for patients coming round from anaesthesia after surgery. You will stay in this room, still watched over by monitoring equipment, until you are fully awake and ready to be returned to your own ward.

If you are in pain when you wake up, tell a nurse in the recovery room as you can be given an injection or tablets to relieve it.

Back on the ward

If you are not going home on the day of your operation, you will be taken back to your own ward. Whether your operation has been done as a day-case or in-patient procedure, you will be visited by the anaesthetist, who will ensure that you are having adequate pain relief and have no ill-effects from your operation. Do tell the anaesthetist if you have any concerns or questions.

In a well-organized day-case unit, the nurse in charge will know when patients can go home, will ensure that they are sufficiently well, have an adult to accompany them and a telephone number to ring if there are any problems, and will confirm that a follow-up appointment has been booked for them.

Side-effects of the anaesthetic

There are side-effects that can occur after anaesthesia, but these do not normally last longer than a couple of days. A sore throat is quite common, and is caused by the dry gases breathed while you are asleep, or by the tube that may have been put down your throat to help you breathe during your operation.

If you feel unwell, or have pain anywhere other than at the site of the wound, do tell the anaesthetist or a nurse on your ward so that the reasons for it can be discovered.

Pain relief

In a day-case unit, providing there are no contraindications, you will be given non-steroidal anti-inflammatory drugs together with analgesics for pain relief. You will also be given a laxative to take home with you, as many analgesics are slightly constipating. For in-patients, particularly after a mastectomy, pethidine or morphine is often given for the first 12-24 hours. However, if these drugs do not adequately relieve your pain, do tell the anaesthetist or ward staff, who may be able to give you something more effective.

The amount of pain suffered after breast surgery varies from person to person. Some women have pain or slight discomfort for only 12-24 hours and will not need any pain-killing injections after this. Others may need injections for up to 3 days after their operation.

Chapter 9

Surgery for breast lumps

Many of the operations for diseases of the breast are relatively simple, causing little trauma. Although almost all breast surgery is done with a general anaesthetic, the surgical approach varies from surgeon to surgeon.

The minor breast operations leave little cosmetic defect, and the incisions used should produce acceptable scars. However, the removal of a breast to treat cancer is a mutilating procedure and the decision to go ahead with this type of surgery is one that is not taken lightly. If you are due to undergo a mastectomy, sufficient time should be allowed for you to receive counselling beforehand and you should be absolutely certain that you understand what is involved. Apart from the mutilation - both physical and psychological - which may be extensive, there may be plans for post-operative chemotherapy and radiotherapy. Therefore, all aspects of these treatments should be explained clearly to you by medical staff, and you should understand them sufficiently to be able to give your fully informed consent. It is a good idea to talk to your breast care nurse about the treatment that is proposed for you at this stage.

Surgery for benign diseases

Fine-needle aspiration cytology and Tru-Cut® biopsy (see pp. 18 and 20) have largely removed the need for excision surgery. However, some women still prefer to have a lump excised and there are occasions when a surgeon feels that excision of a lump (for example an enlarging fibroadenoma, see p. 32) is appropriate.

All breast lumps should be orientated before being sent to the pathology laboratory. This means that they are mounted on a card and the cranial/caudal and medial/lateral parameters as well as the relationship of the lump to the nipple and the axilla are marked. Thus, if the lump is found to be malignant, the pathologist can give a clear indication of the excision margins.

Incisions

Most incisions on the breast can be cosmetically made, particularly if the operation is simply to remove a breast lump. The incision follows the natural crease lines of the skin, known as Langer's lines. If a truly cosmetic crease line cannot be used, the incision can be hidden within the 'bikini bra' line. Incisions can be circumferential or radial on the breast.

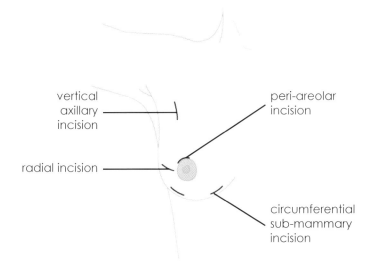

vertical axillary incision

radial incision

peri-areolar incision

circumferential sub-mammary incision

Incisions for breast operations. *Although the exact site of the incision will depend on the position of the lump, this diagram indicates the more common incision sites for the removal of breast lumps.*

Peri-areolar incisions

Incisions made around the pigmented part of the breast allow access to the ducts behind the nipple and to any centrally located breast lumps. Most of these incisions are closed with a subcuticular skin suture (i.e. a stitch beneath the surface of the skin), which is placed from side to side at the skin edges, leaving a fine white line once healing is completed - after about 6 months. There is only a low risk of infection and of cosmetically unacceptable scars following incisions of this type.

Sub-mammary incisions

A sub-mammary incision can be made in the crease underneath the breast to remove the breast completely. The skin and nipple are left intact, together with their blood and nerve supplies. Therefore, sensation is retained (at least partly) in the breast area. An implant can then be placed under the skin, or the breast can be reconstructed in some way (see Chapter 14). Complete removal of the breast by this route is now uncommon and it is certainly not used for operations to treat cancer. It has, however, been used to remove the breast in extreme cases of breast pain.

Biopsy of the breast

Some years ago, surgeons were taught that if a woman had a lump in her breast, the diagnosis should always be confirmed by excision of the lump and examination of it under a microscope. This procedure has now been almost entirely replaced by the use of fine-needle aspiration biopsies or of a wider Tru-Cut® or core biopsy needle (see p. 19). Core biopsy is used to remove a core of breast tissue when a more substantive biopsy is required to allow for a more thorough examination of the architecture of the breast lump.

Although some women would prefer to have a local anaesthetic for an open breast biopsy, this is not usually possible. It is surprisingly difficult, once a small incision has been made in the breast following a local anaesthetic injection, for the surgeon to locate a breast lump, and this is more easily done if a general anaesthetic has been used. Not only is it disconcerting for a surgeon not to be able to find a breast lump that has been hidden by the injection of local anaesthetic, but also the surgeon's concern about the difficulties might be transferred to the patient.

Adair's operation

Also known as Hadfield's operation, this is done to treat duct ectasia (see p. 35).

A general anaesthetic is used and a peri-areolar incision is made around the upper or lower half of the nipple. A small piece of tissue is then removed, which contains the central breast ducts. This tissue is always sent to the pathology laboratory to be looked at under the microscope.

The skin is then closed with a cosmetic subcuticular stitch (also called a suture). The suture is made of either a non-absorbable material such as Prolene (rather like Nylon), which must be taken out after 7-8 days, or an absorbable material that does not need to be removed. There is a tendency for wounds to leak more if closed with the absorbable material, although there is no associated increased risk of infection.

Hadfield's operation has a relatively high incidence of complications, such as haematoma (see p. 95), recurrence of infection, discharge from the wound, retraction of the nipple and a poor cosmetic result. It is not surprising that these complications can occur, given that the operation involves the excision of a 1-cm diameter, 2-3 cm deep cylinder from behind the nipple. However, it is the best operation for recurrent symptomatic duct ectasia, although women having it need good counselling and explanation.

An alternative that is sometimes done is a nipple core biopsy (see p. 19) to remove a section of the breast tissue together with the ducts, which has been found to have a relatively low rate of associated complications.

Microdochectomy

The indication for this operation is a small, warty growth just underneath the nipple and a bloodstained discharge indicative of a papilloma (see p. 34), which may show up on an ultrasound scan.

Under general anaesthesia, the nipple duct is cannulated with a blunt needle and a small triangle of the nipple (including about 4-5 cm of the duct) is removed through a radial incision on the nipple extending to the areola. The tissue specimen is then mounted on a slide and sent for histological examination.

In most cases, the growth is found to be entirely benign. However, if, as happens rarely, an intraductal cancer that is showing some sign of invasion is found, the operation may need to be followed up by more radical surgery.

Surgery for breast cancer

It is very important that women who have been diagnosed as having breast cancer - and their relatives - receive adequate counselling and have time to make an appropriate decision about their treatment. As far as is possible, your surgeon should proceed with your treatment in line with your wishes, having first ensured that you and your family have understood all aspects of the treatment and its implications.

Conservation surgery (i.e. wide local excision, fine-wire local excision biopsy, axillary lymph node sampling and axillary lymph node clearance) can be carried out as a day-case procedure if you are fit and meet the criteria for this type of treatment (see p. 53). If you are having a mastectomy, you may have to stay in hospital until the drainage tubes can be removed, which is usually when less than 40 ml has drained in 24 hours or after 7 days - whichever occurs first. However, even mastectomies are now sometimes done as day-case procedures, allowing women to go home with their drains still in place and to be managed by a district nurse.

There has been a trend over the last few years to move away from the very radical operations performed at the beginning of the twentieth century and well into the 1950s and 1960s. These operations included the removal of not only the breast but also the muscles of the chest wall and all the draining lymph nodes, as it was thought that removing all the lymphatic drainage gave a better chance of cure. With the introduction of radiotherapy and adjuvant therapies such as chemotherapy and with the realization that such radical operations were not necessary for all women, there was a trend towards doing much smaller operations that include conservation of the breast. Nevertheless, there is a very wide spectrum of treatment from a surgeon's point of view. There are, however, three principal operations now performed for breast cancer, all of which are done using a full general anaesthetic.

Wide local excision

Wide local excision involves the removal of the cancerous lump together with a 2-cm (¾-inch) margin of normal breast tissue and usually an ellipse of skin from over the lump. Some lymph nodes are also removed from the armpit for staging (see p. 50), to give an idea of whether the disease has spread beyond the breast. A separate incision may be needed for this. As described on p. 74, once the tumour has been excised, it is orientated on a card and the pathologist gives a full report about the excision margins. A modification of this operation used to be known as a segmental quadrantectomy.

Wide local excision is particularly appropriate for peripheral cancers up to 3 cm in size, depending on the size of the breast. The cosmetic results of the operation are usually good. However, when it is done to remove large tumours in the centre of the breast, it can have very disfiguring cosmetic results. Occasionally, particularly in the upper, inner quadrant of the breast, the incision needs to be made as near to the areola as possible for a good cosmetic result.

The operation alone, with no adjuvant treatment, is associated with a high rate of recurrent cancer in the wound or around the scar. However, it has been shown unequivocally that when combined with 'field' radiotherapy to the remaining breast tissue and to the lymphatic drainage in the armpit, above the collarbone and by the breastbone, it is equivalent to doing a mastectomy. Conservative treatment of this sort can leave a very acceptable cosmetic result, with a normal-looking and normal-feeling breast and nipple.

Simple total mastectomy

In this operation, an ellipse of skin is taken from around the cancer and the nipple. The incision tends to be in line with the nipple and wherever the cancer is. Thus, if the cancer is in the upper, outer quadrant, as is usually the case, the skin ellipse is likely to be in an oblique direction from the armpit, aiming towards the midline. If the lump is to one or other side of the nipple, the incision will be a transverse one.

If too much skin is removed or if the skin flaps are too thin or under tension, the skin that remains may die and there is a risk that a skin graft will be required later. Therefore, only as much skin as necessary is removed. The subcutaneous fat is kept in place to give a cosmetically acceptable scar and to allow for the use of a prosthesis in the bra later. It is uncertain whether leaving more skin to facilitate a later reconstruction of the breast is dangerous in terms of ensuring the removal of all cancerous tissue, but most surgeons will err on the cautious side in any cancer operation.

The whole breast is removed, together with the tail of the breast that goes into the armpit, and its associated lymph nodes. If all the lymph nodes are excised, one of the chest wall muscles (the pectoralis minor muscle) must be split or removed to allow good access to the armpit.

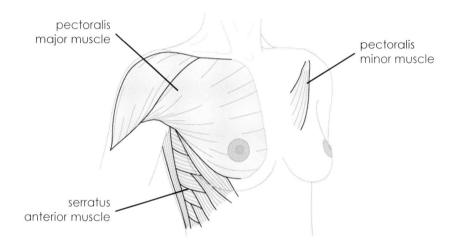

pectoralis major muscle

pectoralis minor muscle

serratus anterior muscle

The chest muscles. *This diagram shows the muscles of the chest wall that may be removed in the more radical mastectomy operations. The pectoralis minor muscle lies beneath the pectoralis major.*

Radiotherapy is not necessarily required, although there is controversy about this. Some surgeons believe that if all the lymph nodes are removed from the armpit, radiotherapy is unnecessary and, indeed, that if it were given, there would be an increased risk of swelling of the arm post-operatively. Others believe that only sampling of the lowest lymph nodes in the armpit is necessary. If the nodes are found not to be involved, it is clear that the cancer is probably confined to the breast and radiotherapy is therefore unnecessary. The decision about which of these two types of treatment to perform is a difficult one, for both the patient and the surgeon, and needs to be discussed carefully.

Axillary lymph node sampling or clearance

Depending on your surgeon's preference and your agreement, assessment of the axillary lymph nodes - which is so important in establishing the prognosis and treatment - is routinely carried out. You should be warned that axillary lymph node sampling is going to be more troublesome to you than the breast surgery itself. This is because the dissection is deeper and often involves the division of the intercostobrachial nerve, which supplies the skin on the side of the upper arm, and you may therefore experience discomfort and swelling due to the collection of lymph and numbness in the axilla and upper arm.

The number of lymph nodes removed together with the degree of lymph node involvement will determine the adjuvant treatment - whether it is radiotherapy for the involved lymph nodes and/or chemotherapy, particularly for younger women.

Sentinel node biopsy

Most breast cancers are now known to spread through the lymphatics in the axilla along a predictable path, the lowermost lymph node (the sentinel node) being affected first. It is rare for breast cancer to spread to axillary lymph nodes higher up in the chain having missed the sentinel node - something that occurs in only about 3% of cases. This discovery has led to the recent introduction of a procedure known as sentinel node biopsy, which provides information about the risk of the cancer recurring.

A dye or radioactive isotope is injected into the axilla to identify the sentinel node - either before or during surgery. When a radioactive isotope is used, the surgeon uses a hand-held gamma-counter to locate the sentinel node. A biopsy is done of the node and, if it is negative (i.e. does not contain malignant cells), it is reasonable to assume that the cancer has not spread to the lymphatics and no sampling of the other lymph nodes is therefore required. If, on the other hand, there are signs of spread of the cancer to the sentinel node, the axillary lymph nodes can be removed.

Chapter 10
After your operation

In hospital

An operation to remove a lump from your breast will probably last about 20-30 minutes; mastectomies may take up to an hour. Therefore, you are likely to be away from the ward for no more than 3-4 hours. When you come round from a general anaesthetic, you may feel drowsy and slightly sick as its effects wear off. If your mouth is dry, you can take sips of water, but drinking too much immediately after your operation can make any nausea worse. As your digestive system will not be affected by the operation, you will be able to eat as soon as you want to.

Following a mastectomy, you may be returned to the ward with a drip inserted into your arm. This contains a saline solution to replace the fluids that have been lost from your body during the operation; it will be removed after about 24 hours or when you are able to drink freely.

Drainage tubes

Drainage tubes may not be necessary, but if they are, one or more small tubes will extend out of the side of the dressing covering your wound, each draining into a plastic bag or bottle, which will probably be placed beside you in the bed. Although the drainage system is cumbersome, you will be able to get up and move around the ward while it is still attached, but do remember to make sure the collecting bag(s) is supported before you do so. The bag may be taped to the side of your body or pinned to your nightdress. The weight of an unsupported bag will pull on the wound, causing discomfort.

During the first day following your operation, fresh blood and fluid will drain into the collecting bag. On the second day, the amount of fluid will probably have reduced substantially and may be mostly clear, with a small amount of blood. Following a wide local excision, the single drainage tube may be removed after about 24 hours. If you do not have a drainage tube, you may be able to go home the day after your operation. Each of the two tubes required after a mastectomy will be taken out when the drainage into them has reduced, which may be after anything from 1 to 7 days.

It is possible to return home with a drainage tube in place after day-case surgery, in which case it will be removed at a hospital visit 1-2 days later.

The wound

Your wound may be covered by a clear dressing, with an overlying pressure dressing to reduce bruising. The pressure dressing consists of a wad of gauze covered with Elastoplast strapping, which is quite tightly applied after wide local excisions and mastectomies. This dressing will probably be removed after about 24 hours, once a doctor has visited you on the ward to check your wound.

If you do not want to be able to see the wound through the remaining clear adhesive dressing, do ask a nurse to cover it with gauze. You may find the sight of the blood-encrusted wound, the stitches and possibly bruising upsetting. However, it will improve each day and it should have healed and begun to look a lot better after a couple of weeks.

Your wound may have been stitched with an absorbable material that will dissolve of its own accord in time and therefore does not need to be removed. Only the ends of absorbable stitches may be visible; the ends of non-absorbable stitches may have a small, white bead attached. Some surgeons prefer to use stitches made of a non-absorbable material, as they feel that these result in a better scar. Stitches of this type will have to be removed 7-14 days after surgery. Many wounds are now stitched with a single continuous stitch and appear as a single line.

The pull of the stitches may cause a feeling of tightness, which will improve after a few days.

Painkillers

A local anaesthetic may have been injected, as a nerve block or into the wound during your operation, to reduce the pain as you regain consciousness (see p. 70). Its effects should last for about 6-8 hours. After this, and while you are still in hospital, you will be able to have pain-killing tablets, or injections if necessary. Do ask for these injections if you need them, although they are rarely required because the pain level following this type of surgery is not normally high and regular oral analgesic tablets such as aspirin, paracetamol or Nurofen will probably be enough. Make sure you have some of these tablets at home for the next few days. Painkillers should be taken regularly (every 4-6 hours, or as indicated on their container) so that their effect does not wear off before you take the next dose. A dose as you go to bed may help relieve any discomfort and allow you to get a good night's sleep.

If you have had axillary lymph glands removed, your armpit may be sore for a few days and possibly numb for several weeks or months.

Getting out of bed

Effective pain control enables you to get out of bed and to move around with ease soon after your operation, usually on the day after surgery. Movement and exercise are important to avoid deep vein thrombosis (see p. 94) and to keep your bladder and lungs working properly.

You should be able to get up and walk about as soon as the anaesthetic effects wear off. Once you are fully mobile, you will be able to remove your anti-embolism stockings (see p. 63).

Bra padding

Before you leave hospital, you will be fitted with a temporary pad (see p. 110) to put in your bra if you have lost a part or the whole of your breast. The pad will give some shape to your affected breast and will also help to protect your wound. It can be worn at night if desired. Once the wound has healed, a more permanent prosthesis will be fitted if you want one (see p. 110).

Shoulder movement

Immediately after your operation, you may have limited shoulder movement, but your range of shoulder movements should gradually return to normal within 2-4 weeks with gentle exercising.

A physiotherapist may visit you on the ward the day after your operation to assess your degree of shoulder movement. You will also be advised about exercises to help you regain the normal range of movement of the arm and shoulder on your affected side (see below) and you may be given a leaflet explaining how to do them. *It is important to follow the specific instructions you are given about when and how to exercise.*

There are some very simple exercises you can do while still in hospital to help prevent stiffness developing in your arm and shoulder. For example, you can use your good arm to assist your affected arm with upward and sideways movements, and can try to brush your hair with your elbow resting on a table. Once you are at home again, you should exercise your arm and shoulder while carrying out your normal daily routine, for example while dusting and doing light housework.

Although the muscles in the chest wall are now not usually removed during a mastectomy unless they are involved in the tumour, they can become weakened by under-use after this operation. Exercises to help regain muscle strength are therefore also important.

Discomfort following a mastectomy may also cause you to change your posture, for example by leaning towards the side of discomfort or bending forward. Good posture is important so that back pain does not become a problem.

Exercises

You will be given a leaflet while in hospital giving advice about which exercises to do and how often to do them. The exercises are designed to help you extend your range of movement and to prevent shoulder problems developing, which can cause pain and restricted arm movement.

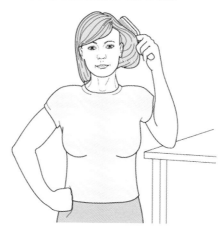

Brushing your hair. *A simple exercise to help regain shoulder movement after surgery.*

For the first few days you may experience some discomfort while doing the exercises, but if they become too painful, you should stop and try again gently later.

The following are some general exercises that may be helpful, but do follow the specific advice given to you by your physiotherapist.

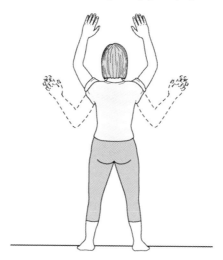

Exercise 1 *Stand facing a wall with your feet apart so that you are well balanced. Place your hands on the wall, level with your shoulders, and work them slowly upwards as far as is comfortable. Slide your hands back to shoulder level and repeat the exercise, trying to get a bit higher each time.*

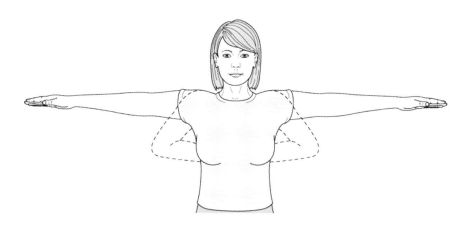

Exercise 2 *Stand with your arms stretched out to the sides and level with your shoulders. Slowly bring them down and behind your back until they reach to bra level.*

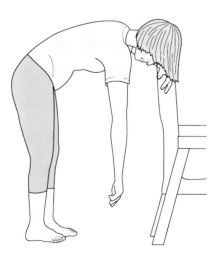

Exercise 3 *Standing at arm's length from a chair, hold the back of the chair with the hand on your unaffected side and rest your forehead on this arm. Hang your other arm loosely down and swing it gently from the shoulder, backwards and forwards, from side to side, and then in small circles, gradually increasing the size of the swings and circles as you feel able to do so.*

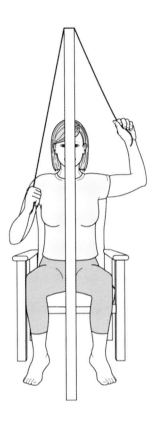

Exercise 4 *Hang a rope or piece of cord over the top of an open door and sit on a chair with the door between your legs. Holding the lower end of the rope in the hand on your affected side, gently pull the other end so that your affected arm is raised as high as possible without causing too much discomfort. Gradually increase the amount you raise your affected arm as the movement returns to your shoulder.*

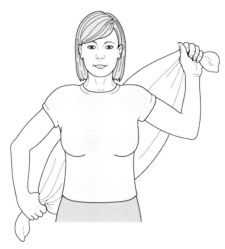

Exercise 5 *Hold a towel diagonally across your back and move it as though you are drying yourself. Then repeat the exercise with the towel held diagonally the other way.*

Going home

Some time after your operation, a hospital doctor will visit you on the ward to check that all is well. Before you are discharged from hospital, the nursing staff will need to be sure you will be able to manage. If you do not have help at home and are concerned about managing on your own, do tell one of the nurses before your operation so that some arrangement can be made for you. For some people, such as elderly women who live on their own, a longer stay in hospital may be necessary until they are better able to cope.

By the time you are discharged from hospital you should have only slight pain or discomfort, your wound will be healing and any drains will probably have been removed.

Driving

You should not drive yourself home after your operation and should probably avoid driving for at least 2 weeks. Your car insurance is likely to be invalid for at least 48 hours after a general anaesthetic: you may feel all right, but your reactions in an emergency would be slower than normal.

Even if you have not had a general anaesthetic, do not drive until you are sure you can make an emergency stop without being hindered by pain from your wound. If you are in any doubt, your family doctor will be able to advise you about this.

Discharge letter

Before you leave hospital, you will be given a letter to take to your family doctor. This will contain a report of the operation and anything your doctor may need to know about your treatment. The letter may be posted to your doctor if you leave hospital before it has been written.

Follow-up clinic visits

Before you leave the hospital, nursing staff will arrange your next clinic visit - within a week or two of your operation. Time will be allowed for the results to be received from the examination of your breast tissue that always follows an operation on the breast.

If the stitches in your wound are non-absorbable, they will either be removed at the clinic visit or, if nursing staff think your wound will have healed sufficiently beforehand, you will be asked to make an appointment for them to be removed at your health centre or doctor's surgery.

Although the anxiety you and your family will feel while you await this next visit to the clinic is well understood by the nursing and medical staff, they must be sure that the results from the laboratory will have been received first.

The doctor will examine you, but do make sure you mention any problems you are having, such as difficulty in extending your arm.

Visit from the breast care nurse

If your hospital has a specialist breast care nurse (see p. 21), she will visit you on the ward before you leave. Do tell her if you are concerned about anything or if there is anything you do not understand. She may be able to arrange a date to visit you at home, if you would like her to do so, and will probably continue to see you as often as necessary, either at home or in her clinic. Most breast care nurses provide a post-discharge service for one-to-one sessions that give women time to talk about how they feel and about the impact their treatment has had on them.

At home

You may have some pain or discomfort in your breast or across your chest at the operation site for a few days. Any numbness or 'tingling' sensation under your arm may last several weeks or months. If you have had a mastectomy or axillary lymph glands removed, your shoulder will probably also be stiff. The exercises explained above will help you to regain the movement in your arm and, apart from doing these regularly, you should try to use your arm normally as much as possible. However, heavy housework and lifting should be avoided for about 6 weeks and you should use your other arm to carry shopping etc.

Anxiety and depression

You will probably feel tired for at least a few days and may find you become easily depressed. Many women experience a sense of elation immediately after their operation, which then gives way to lethargy and exhaustion as the anxiety they have been feeling starts to be relieved. Mood swings are common, ranging from elation to depression and anger. This is a normal reaction, which should settle down in time.

It is also common for anxiety to return 2-3 months after surgery, but the majority of women are able to develop coping skills and to go on to live a normal life. However, for some women, depression or sexual problems continue for many months, and it is important for them to talk to their doctor or breast care nurse about these so that arrangements can be made for any necessary counselling or other treatment. The persistence of this sort of problem does not seem to be related to the type of operation that has been done, and women who have had conservative surgery are just as likely to become anxious and depressed as those who have undergone mastectomy. Mastectomy can lead to concerns about body image and loss of femininity, and some women worry that they will be less attractive to their partners, or will be unable to find a partner, after a breast operation, although in the majority of cases these fears are unfounded. Women who have had conservative surgery may be equally worried about the possibility of the cancer recurring. Again, do discuss your concerns with your breast care nurse. There are also numerous support groups for women with breast cancer, and a list of those in your area can be obtained from the organizations listed in Appendix IV.

If you have problems sleeping and are waking up in the night and worrying so that you are exhausted during the day, your family doctor should be able to prescribe a light sedative for you to take for a few nights. Even three good nights' sleep can help you to cope again and can stop the cycle of tiredness and anxiety.

If your appetite is poor, it will improve in time and you should eat what you want when you want until it does so.

Although you should take things easy and rest when you need to for the first few days you are at home, it is important to try to get out and about as much as possible and to return to your normal life as soon as you feel able to do so.

Telling children about cancer

Young children can only understand very simple explanations about why their mothers have had to go into hospital. By the age of 10, most children can grasp quite complicated details and it is better to be honest rather than let their imaginations dream up something much worse than the reality. However, it is probably better to give them a little information at a time and to build up the whole picture gradually, taking your cue from your children about how much they want to know. All children need reassurance and a chance to express their own fears and talk about things if they want to. Older children may find their anxieties difficult to cope with and to express or understand. They should be encouraged to talk about their fears, but not pushed into doing so before they are ready.

Chapter 11

Post-operative complications

As with any type of operation, there can be general complications following breast surgery, such as chest infection and deep vein thrombosis (see below). Although minor complications are fairly common, serious ones are rare. If you are at all concerned about anything that occurs after your operation, contact your doctor, the consultant or the hospital ward for advice. Although serious complications are not common, it is better to err on the safe side and most doctors will be happy to discuss your worries with you.

Poor posture can lead to back pain, and reduced mobility and strength in the shoulder are sometimes caused by the adhesion of muscle fibres following breast operations. Nerve damage during surgery can also lead to problems such as restricted arm movement, making it difficult, for example, to carry a book under your arm. Good physiotherapy advice and regular exercises can help prevent or alleviate these complications.

General complications

Chest infections

Chest infections can occur following general anaesthesia for any type of operation and particularly when a painful wound makes deep breathing more difficult. They are especially common in smokers. Deep breathing is important after your operation to keep the lungs well aerated. If you find it difficult, a physiotherapist may be able to visit you on the ward to advise you about breathing exercises.

Pneumothorax

Very rarely, when the breast and underlying muscles are removed, it is possible for the membrane between the ribs to be damaged, thus allowing air to enter the thoracic cavity. This rare condition (known as pneumothorax) can cause partial or total collapse of the lungs. An X-ray of the chest may be taken following a radical mastectomy to make sure that this type of damage has not occurred.

If you cough up blood and have a pain in your chest following a radical mastectomy, you should tell your doctor so that the possibility of a pneumothorax can be investigated.

Deep vein thrombosis

This is quite a common complication following pelvic surgery, but less so after other types of operation. Precautions such as wearing anti-embolism stockings while immobile (see p. 63) and having a course of heparin injections (see p. 63) are usually taken to help prevent it occurring. If a blood clot (thrombus) forms in the deep veins of the body - most commonly in the calf veins of the legs - it can break away and the resulting embolus may pass through the heart and block the arteries of the lungs. The resulting *pulmonary embolism* can be life threatening. If a thrombus is detected, it can be treated with a course of heparin or warfarin.

Pyrexia

Pyrexia is simply fever, which can occur during the first 24 hours after an operation. The cause of a persistent or high fever may need to be investigated; it is most likely to be a chest or wound infection or deep vein thrombosis. However, starting deep breathing exercises as soon as possible after surgery can help to prevent fever developing, and deep breathing can also sometimes correct a fever once it has developed.

Local complications

Pain and bruising

Local anaesthetic will probably be injected into the skin edges prior to closing the wound to help reduce the pain once you wake up. This pain-killing effect lasts for several hours, but when it wears off, you will need another form of pain relief for a while.

A sharp, intermittent pain in the chest wall is probably due to nerve regeneration or a trapped nerve, whereas an aching pain in the anterior chest can be caused by spasm of the pectoralis major muscle. Pain in the upper arm may be referred from the spine, possibly resulting from bad posture, or if the pain is in the back of the upper arm, it can be due to nerve regeneration.

A stabbing pain may occur in the upper, outer part of the arm and is likely to be associated with the return of sensation to the arm as post-operative numbness wears off. This type of pain may not develop until a week or two after your operation.

Persistent pain that is not relieved by painkillers such as paracetamol, although unlikely to have a serious cause, is worth investigating and you should seek medical advice if it occurs.

Even minor breast operations can cause severe bruising, which can be extensive and last for several days or weeks. Although this type of severe bruising may be distressing to look at, there is unlikely to be any cause for concern.

Haematoma

A haematoma is a collection of blood that leaks from the tissues during or after an operation and is unable to escape. Blood may collect under the skin flaps that remain after a breast operation, although this is uncommon, as the surgeon will have taken care to stop bleeding during surgery. The drainage tubes that are inserted into the breast are left in place until there is no further seepage of blood or fluid. Rarely, a haematoma may need to be removed by means of a simple, short operation.

Wound infection

Infection can occur in the breast wound, which will become red, hard and tender, possibly discharging pus if an abscess has formed. Wound infection can cause fever and sweating and may make you feel generally unwell. Abscesses can normally be treated effectively by releasing the pus they contain and by a course of antibiotics.

When a large area of skin has been removed, and the remaining skin flaps cannot be pulled together easily, a skin graft may be necessary to fill the gap. If the edges of the skin flaps are pulled together too tightly, they may die and healing can be delayed. It is also possible (but rare) for more extensive skin damage to develop if the blood supply to the edges of the skin is cut off. The skin may turn black (gangrene) or it may swell and become inflamed. If this occurs, immediate treatment will be necessary to reverse the gangrene or to prevent it worsening.

Fluid collection

Fluid collection is common following wide local excisions and mastectomies. The fluid may need to be aspirated repeatedly and the condition can be extremely uncomfortable. Do seek your doctor's advice as soon as possible if fluid collects quickly after aspiration.

The skin flaps often become raised by a collection of fluid that forms a *seroma*, which can develop despite the use of drains to withdraw fluid from the operation site. Some fluid probably comes from the lymphatics and from the bare muscle exposed when a breast has been removed. The fluid is usually a light, golden colour and is not bloody. Although seromas can be persistent, the collected fluid can simply be drawn off with a needle, which is inserted painlessly through the scar.

Lymphoedema

Water and protein leak constantly from the blood vessels and tissues of the body and are drained away in the lymphatic vessels. A network of small lymphatic vessels links up with deeper, larger ones in the groin and under the arms and it is at these sites that the lymph is filtered through lymph nodes (or glands), before being returned to the bloodstream. When the lymph nodes are removed, or the lymphatic vessels are damaged during a breast operation, the lymph may not be able to drain away, and swelling (known as lymphoedema) of the arm may occur. When lymphoedema does develop, it is difficult to treat.

Symptoms and signs

Lymphoedema can be a severe and sometimes extremely debilitating condition. The first signs of it - for example tightening of a watch strap or rings - should be reported to your doctor or breast care nurse immediately, because early treatment has a better chance of being effective.

Redness and soreness of the arm may be signs of infection of the surface tissues (cellulitis) and, if they develop, they will require early treatment with antibiotics. Infection in a swollen arm may be followed by a blood clot and inflammation of a vein (a condition known as thrombo-phlebitis). It is therefore important to take care to avoid injury to the arm on the affected side of your body.

A swollen arm can cause discomfort and a feeling of tightness, but if you develop any of the following symptoms or signs, you should contact your doctor:

❖ numbness or pins and needles in a swollen arm,

❖ sharp, stabbing pains,

❖ a burning sensation or extreme tenderness,

❖ weakness in the arm or a sudden inability to grip.

Treatment

Although lymphoedema cannot be cured once it has developed, the arm-raising exercises described in Chapter 10 can help to reduce the swelling and prevent it getting worse. Lymphoedema may be controlled by a combination of regular, gentle exercise, massage (which you will have to be taught), general skin care and, when appropriate, by the wearing of an elastic compression sleeve. Although you can carry out most of the measures to control lymphoedema yourself, you must ask your doctor's advice before starting any form of treatment.

Preventing infection and injury

Germs can enter the body through dry, cracked skin and you should therefore use a simple moisturizer after every bath. If your skin has become very rough, your doctor will be able to prescribe a special cream to treat it.

You should always protect the hand and arm on your affected side from injury and possible infection, for example by wearing gloves while you are gardening or using strong cleansing agents and by using a thimble when sewing. If your hand or arm is cut or grazed, however small the injury, make sure it is thoroughly cleaned, treated with antiseptic and covered with a clean dressing. If persistent inflammation or swelling follows an injury of this sort, ask your doctor's advice as soon as possible.

Blood pressure measurement, blood tests and injections should be done on the other arm whenever possible.

Movement and exercise

Gravity tends to cause the lymph to pool and its effect can be counteracted by raising the arm whenever possible. Your affected arm should be rested on a cushion (on the arm of a chair when sitting and beside you when you are in bed) so that it is above the level of your heart.

Although too much exercise will cause the swelling to increase, gentle, regular movement of the arm helps the lymphatic fluid to drain away. The exercises described above should be done gently, at least once a day, while wearing a compression sleeve if you have one (see below).

Massage

Massage of the affected arm and armpit, as well as of the lymph glands in the neck, will help lymphatic drainage away from the arm. Massage clears the way ahead of the swelling so that fluid can drain from the swollen area. It should be gentle but firm, just enough to move the skin. It is important that the massage is done correctly to aid lymph drainage, and a nurse or physiotherapist should be able to show you how to do it.

Compression sleeves

In some cases of lymphoedema, an elastic compression sleeve may be worn, which prevents fluid building up in the arm and provides support to the muscles. These sleeves can be obtained from a hospital appliance officer, to whom you must be referred by your consultant or breast care nurse.

Compression sleeves should be put on in the morning when the swelling is least and can be removed at night. Moist skin makes them more difficult to apply and it is therefore best not to have a bath immediately before fitting your sleeve. Once the sleeve is on, it should be smooth and creaseless. It should never be rolled back, because it will act as a tourniquet. The elastic gradually loses its strength and the sleeve will need to be replaced every 3-4 months.

It is important that you wear your elastic sleeve in hot weather, even though it may be uncomfortable, as this is a time when your arm is likely to swell.

Compression pumps

The use of a compression pump (Flowtron®) is not suitable in every case; your doctor will be able to advise you about this. The pump is attached by a small tube to an inflatable cuff and is powered from the mains electricity. Air is pumped in to inflate the cuff and is then gradually sucked out to deflate it again. The effect is a gentle squeezing of the arm, which assists the drainage of lymph away from it. Compression pumps are normally used at regular intervals throughout the day to help reduce swelling.

Your pump should not be used if you have an infection in your arm or swelling in your chest or if it causes pain.

If you are attending a lymphoedema clinic, your progress will be regularly monitored and you will be given advice about all the measures you can take to help control the condition.

Other complications

As has already been mentioned (see p. 69), there is always a small risk associated with the use of a general anaesthetic. However, you are far more likely to be run over while crossing the road than to suffer any serious complication caused by a general anaesthetic.

Very rarely, the supply of oxygen to the brain can be interrupted during anaesthesia, and brain damage (possibly with paralysis) or death can occur. Although this risk has to be borne in mind, it is extremely rare and should be kept in perspective.

Other minor complications of general anaesthesia are a sore throat, cough and chest infection. Muscle pain, which may develop as a result of the muscle relaxants used, usually lasts for no more than 48 hours.

Recurrence

One of the worst complications to follow surgery for cancer is to have a recurrence of the disease. The risk of cancer recurring in the scar of the operation or in the lymphatics in the armpit is around 1%. The surgeon will take all possible steps to be sure that local control of the cancer is achieved. Recurrence outside the area of the breast and its immediate lymphatic drainage is less easy to predict and to treat.

If recurrence of breast cancer is suspected, it is important for staging to take place (see p. 50). A blood test will be done, as well as a chest X-ray, isotope bone scan and ultrasound scan of the liver to look for metastases (see p. 49).

Chapter 12
Hormone therapy, radiotherapy & chemotherapy

Adjuvant therapy

Following surgery for breast cancer, you may be referred to a cancer specialist (an oncologist) for further treatment. Treatment that is done in addition to the main form of treatment - in this case surgery - is known as adjuvant therapy. Its aim in treating women with breast cancer is to destroy any cancer cells that may remain in the body after the tumour has been surgically removed or to reduce the tumour in size before surgery.

Following an operation for breast cancer, the adjuvant therapy may be with hormones (endocrine therapy), X-rays (radiotherapy) or drugs (chemotherapy). You will see a consultant in clinical or medical oncology and may be given one of these forms of treatment or a combination of any of them. You may receive the adjuvant treatment at the same hospital at which your operation was done, or you may have to go to a cancer centre at another hospital.

Some time before your treatment starts, the oncologist will examine you and look at the results of your operation and of any investigations that have been done. Occasionally, further investigations are needed, such as a liver or bone scan, to determine whether the cancer has spread beyond your breast. The oncologist will then discuss the proposed treatment plan with you and you will be able to ask questions.

Hormone therapy

It has long been recognized that the female hormone oestrogen can stimulate the growth of breast cancer. Most oestrogen is produced by the ovaries until they cease to function at menopause. Even after the menopause, some oestrogen is still produced by the adrenal glands.

Clinical trials

To be able to improve the treatment given to women with breast cancer, new drugs need to be tested and currently used drugs and radiotherapy regimes need to be tried in different ways. Therefore, many women are asked to take part in clinical trials to compare a new treatment with an existing one.

If your specialist is involved in a trial of this sort, you may be asked if you would be willing to take part. The details of the trial will be explained to you and you should make sure you fully understand what is entailed before you make a decision. You are under no obligation to agree to be involved and, if you refuse, the quality of the treatment you receive will not be affected in any way.

Studies have indicated that women who take part in clinical trials tend to do better than those who do not participate, and therefore it is worth finding out as much as you can about any clinical trial you are invited to be involved in and to give serious consideration to taking part. Do talk over the pros and cons with your family doctor to help you make your decision.

Tamoxifen

The most common hormone treatment is tamoxifen. It is given by mouth and blocks the action of oestrogen on breast cancer cells, thus preventing them growing and multiplying. It will also act against breast cancer cells that may have spread to other parts of the body before the breast cancer was removed surgically.

The many trials that have been carried out to assess the use of tamoxifen have shown it to be of benefit to almost all women with breast cancer. Although a cure cannot be guaranteed, tamoxifen does significantly reduce the risk of the cancer recurring. It has maximum benefit in the first 2 years of its use, and it is therefore usual to limit the course of this drug to 5 years. It is particularly effective in post-menopausal women and in those with oestrogen-receptor-positive tumours.

Side-effects of tamoxifen

Although tamoxifen can cause side-effects in some women, its benefits for women with breast cancer far outweigh any risks associated with it - and it also protects against osteoporosis and heart disease.

The most common side-effects (which occur in about 30% of women) include mild weight gain, sweats and flushing, which tend to reduce in time but which may require specific therapy and sometimes withdrawal of the drug. It can also cause vaginal dryness, irritation and pain during intercourse (dyspareunia). These effects are due to vaginal atrophy, which may result from the lack of oestrogen caused by tamoxifen, and can be treated with oestrogen in the form of pessaries or cream, which is only minimally absorbed. Thrush (an infection caused by fungi of the species *Candida*) is also common.

Intermenstrual or post-coital bleeding or heavy, prolonged bleeding should be reported to your general practitioner, who will arrange for you to be referred to a gynaecologist for investigation.

Prolonged treatment with tamoxifen leads to patchy endometrial hyperplasia, dysplasia and eventually carcinoma *in situ* and invasive carcinoma of the body of the uterus in a small percentage of women who have taken the drug for more than 10 years.

Other hormone therapies

In pre-menopausal women, endocrine treatment used to involve the removal of the ovaries in an operation called oophorectomy or by radiation treatment. However, these procedures are increasingly being replaced by the use of hormone analogues that block oestrogen secretion. Hormone treatment is also given to post-menopausal women to delay the progression of breast cancer and to improve its symptoms.

Goserelin (Zoladex) is antagonistic to the output from the pituitary of follicle-stimulating hormone (FSH) and luteinizing hormone (I H), both of which stimulate the ovaries. It is given as monthly injections. When treatment with goserelin stops, normal menstrual periods are restored. Its prolonged use can, however, lead to osteoporosis.

Megestrol (Megace) is a progestogen (see p.55), which is also effective in the treatment of breast cancer, but can cause considerable weight gain.

Anastrozole (Arimidex) is an aromatase inhibitor that interferes with the production of the sex hormones, both in the ovary and in the adrenal glands. Its use is particularly appropriate for post-menopausal women, but it is also gaining favour as a first-line treatment instead of tamoxifen.

Radiotherapy

Radiotherapy involves directing high-energy X-ray beams at specific areas of the body. The procedure is painless and is similar to having a normal X-ray taken, except the radiation dose is higher and exposure to it lasts a couple of minutes rather than a fraction of a second. The cosmetic appearance following radiotherapy is usually reasonably good.

Cancer cells are more sensitive than normal cells and are therefore selectively destroyed by the radiation directed at them. As radiotherapy is given after the tumour mass has been surgically removed, the radiation is only required to destroy any remaining microscopic cancer. You will need to have radiotherapy if you have undergone conservative surgery (see p. 55), and the glands under your arm and at the side of your neck may also be treated.

It is not usually necessary to have radiotherapy following a mastectomy, unless the tumour was large or the cancer cells had spread to a number of lymph nodes. In these cases, the area around the mastectomy scar, and possibly the draining lymph nodes, may be treated in an attempt to destroy any cancer cells that may not have been removed surgically.

Once you have undergone radiotherapy, it may not be possible for you to have this type of treatment again if the cancer recurs in your breast, chest wall, mastectomy scar or axillary lymph nodes.

Pre-treatment appointment

Before your treatment starts, you will be given an appointment to meet the radiographers who will give you your radiotherapy and the radiotherapist or oncologist who will supervise it. You will be asked to lie on the treatment couch and marks will be made on your skin to indicate where the X-ray beam should be directed. It is important that some of these marks remain until your course of treatment has finished and you should therefore be careful not to wash them off if you have a bath. In fact, the radiotherapist may tell you to keep the treatment area completely dry for the duration of your treatment and until any skin reaction has settled down. The marks may also leave traces on your undergarments and it is advisable not to wear a new or special bra until after your course of treatment.

Measurements will be taken of your breast or chest and an outline of your body will be drawn. These preparations are to make sure you are placed in the correct position every time you receive treatment.

Receiving the treatment

Radiotherapy is usually given after chemotherapy and is not usually started until at least 8 weeks following surgery. This delay also allows time for your wound to heal and for movement to be regained in your arm, so that it can be raised above your head and thus placed outside the field of treatment.

The course of radiotherapy will probably last 4-6 weeks, with sessions daily or every other day. Although the length of the treatment sessions may vary from centre to centre, each one normally takes about 15-20 minutes, most of which time is spent getting you into the correct position.

You will be alone in the room during exposure to the radiation, but will be watched carefully at all times.

Side-effects

Radiotherapy does not make you radioactive and you do not need to avoid close contact with people after it. It will, however, make you tired and your skin is likely to become sensitive and possibly red and uncomfortable towards the end of your course of treatment. Some women have more sensitive skins than others, and you will be given advice about skin care. If necessary, creams can be prescribed for you if your skin becomes moist and painful.

The area being treated should not be vigorously washed or dried, because this could damage the already tender skin. However, your radiotherapist may agree to you splashing the area with water and patting it dry. Perfume-free talcum powder, such as baby powder, can be used if desired.

If you do have a skin reaction, it should subside within a few weeks once the treatment is finished. Your skin may remain a darker colour for many months and the treated area should be protected from sunlight for at least a year.

Other side-effects following radiotherapy are rare. You will not lose your hair and are unlikely to feel sick. However, the treated breast may remain swollen for anything up to 4 years and will probably occasionally be sore, but any soreness and discomfort may be reduced by anti-inflammatory drugs.

The X-rays could also reach a small part of the lung beneath the breast. Very occasionally, this causes inflammation, with breathlessness and a dry cough, which may not develop for a month or two after the end of your treatment and may last for a few weeks. Lymphoedema may occur if radiotherapy is given after a large number of lymph glands have been surgically removed (see p. 96).

Most women who go out to work are able to continue to do so, at least part time, during their course of radiation treatment.

Chemotherapy

Chemotherapy is rarely administered to women over the age of 70, but it is particularly appropriate for younger women, for whom it is associated with a reduction in recurrence and an improvement in prognosis. Younger women with undifferentiated primary breast cancer (ductal grade III - see p. 50) are most likely to benefit from chemotherapy, as are those with vessel permeation and extensive axillary lymphatic involvement (e.g. seven or eight lymph nodes) and with certain types of tumour.

You may be advised to have chemotherapy if it is thought that there is a high risk of the cancer spreading beyond your breast or its surrounding lymph glands following surgery.

Whereas radiotherapy attacks cancer cells in the specific area at which the X-ray beam is directed, the drugs used in chemotherapy can kill cancer cells throughout the body.

Each woman is assessed individually and the most suitable combination of drugs, the timing and duration of treatment are decided upon. The most commonly prescribed drugs are epirubicin, doxorubicin, cyclophosphamide, methotrexate and fluorouracil. The typical combinations used are:

❖ CMF - cyclophosphamide, methotrexate and fluorouracil,

❖ FEC - fluorouracil, epirubicin and cisplatin.

A group of drugs called the taxanes, which include the newer drugs paclitaxel (Taxol) and docetaxel (Taxotere), and the antibody trastuzumab (Herceptin) are currently being assessed in clinical trials for the treatment of breast cancer. Early results of these trials indicate a considerable benefit associated with the use of the taxanes in primary treatment and of Herceptin in selected patient groups.

Receiving the treatment

You will be given the drugs approximately monthly, by injection or as a combination of injections and tablets. A blood sample will be taken for a blood count before the drugs are administered through a needle inserted into a vein in the back of your hand or forearm. The injections take about 5-10 minutes to administer. Adjuvant chemotherapy is usually given in an out-patient clinic over a period of 4-6 months.

Side-effects

Different drugs have different side-effects, which will be explained to you before your treatment begins. The most common side-effects are nausea, tiredness and effects on the blood count. Some drugs cause extensive hair loss, whereas others cause little or none.

All the side-effects will stop as soon as your course of chemotherapy comes to an end. Any hair that has been lost will grow back as thick as it was before, although the new hair may be a different colour or have changed to become straight or curly.

Do discuss any side-effects you experience with the doctor or nurse, as it may be possible for you to take something to improve the symptoms.

The ovaries

For pre-menopausal women who have a high risk of breast cancer spreading to other parts of their body, it may be advisable to stop their ovaries producing oestrogen. The ovaries can be removed surgically in an operation called bilateral oophorectomy (see p. 43), which can be done either as an open operation or laparoscopically ('keyhole' surgery). Alternatively, the ovaries can be removed by radiotherapy, in which case the change is more gradual. Radiotherapy is usually given over a period of a week and will gradually stop the ovaries working over the next few months.

Advanced disease

For some women, chemotherapy or radiotherapy is used as a primary treatment rather than as an adjuvant following surgery. In the case of a rapidly growing breast cancer, for example, by the time a diagnosis is made the tumour may be too large to be removed surgically, or cancer cells may already have spread to other parts of the body. Therefore, although a biopsy may be done to examine the tumour, the first line of treatment may be chemotherapy or radiotherapy.

Primary chemotherapy

The drugs used are the same as those mentioned above for adjuvant chemotherapy, but they may be given more often or in higher doses.

Your treatment may be administered while you are in hospital or in an out-patient clinic. The doctor will monitor your chemotherapy carefully and will examine you regularly to make sure that the tumour is shrinking. Once the tumour has been reduced to a more manageable size, it may then be removed surgically, followed by a course of radiotherapy.

Primary chemotherapy is used most commonly for young women with large, fast-growing breast cancers, for whom surgery is less mutilating once the size of the tumour has been reduced.

Primary radiotherapy

Again, radiotherapy may be used as primary treatment for a large tumour before it is removed surgically. The course of treatment is longer than that given following surgery, and the radiotherapy may be administered by X-ray beam as well as internally through radioactive wires, which are inserted into the breast under anaesthetic. Some types of radiation treatment are administered in hospital over 3-4 days.

Palliative therapy

When breast cancer is very advanced and cannot be cured, chemotherapy and radiotherapy can be used to slow its growth or help relieve its symptoms. Hormones other than tamoxifen may also be used to slow the growth of a tumour without causing too many side-effects.

Palliative treatment may successfully prevent the cancer from growing for many months or years, even though it cannot be completely eradicated.

Chapter 13

Prostheses

For women who do not want to undergo breast reconstruction (see Chapter 14), but who want to restore the natural outline of a partially or totally removed breast, a wide range of artificial breasts (known as prostheses) is available. Breast prostheses are worn inside the bra and can be matched to the other breast to make it indistinguishable in terms of size and shape.

Temporary prostheses

Immediately following surgery, you can wear a light, temporary prosthesis, which will not press on your wound as it heals. A breast care or other specialist nurse will probably help you to choose and fit a prosthesis of this type before you leave hospital.

The commonly used breast shapes are washable and have a lightweight fibre filling, which can be added to or removed to make them the correct size. They are simply placed inside the bra, which should be as good a fit as possible so that the breast shape remains in place. Safety pins or press studs sewn on to the prosthesis and the inside of the bra cup will also help to prevent the shape becoming dislodged as you move.

Permanent prostheses

Some 6-8 weeks after your operation, or following your course of radiotherapy if you have one, a heavier, permanent prosthesis can be fitted to match the size, shape and weight of your other breast. These prostheses are made from silicone and have a skin-like texture. Although a silicone breast shape can be placed in a cotton cover, which can be removed for washing, it is more often left uncovered so that it can mould to the contours of your chest wall. However, a cover may be useful if the prosthesis becomes uncomfortable or when you are hot.

Some manufacturers make tinted prostheses for women with darker skins; your breast care nurse should be able to advise you about how to select the right one for your skin colour.

All the permanent prostheses have a nipple outline, but it is now also possible to have a separate textured and pigmented nipple and areola, which are also available in a variety of skin tones. The nipple may be attached permanently or semi-permanently to the breast form. Although the artificial nipples look very realistic, they cannot retract and become erect, and there are now nipples available that can be placed over the nipple of the other breast so that the two match.

If you do not have large breasts, you can wear a self-supporting prosthesis that simply sticks to your chest wall. Modern self-supporting prostheses allow complete freedom of movement and will stay in place while you play sport, such as tennis, horse-riding and swimming. Sports bras are only normally necessary for any particularly vigorous sporting activity. This type of prosthesis is useful for women who do not usually wear a bra and for those who like to wear strapless dresses.

The silicone that gives the breast shape bulk and form may be heavy for women with large breasts. Although pads worn under the bra straps may help to take some of the weight off the shoulders, a lighter prosthesis can be used if necessary, for example one with a silicone front. If you have any problems of this sort, your breast care nurse should be able to sort them out for you.

It is quite all right to swim when wearing a silicone prosthesis, as it should not be affected by sea water or the chlorine in a swimming pool. However, it is probably advisable to rinse it in tap water and dry it afterwards.

Silicone prostheses do not usually cause skin irritation, but, very rarely, there can be an allergic reaction to the breast forms, although skin irritation is more likely to be due to a sweat rash. If your skin does appear to be affected, contact your breast care nurse for advice.

Take your time when making your choice of prosthesis. There is a wide variety available and you should be able to find exactly the right one, particularly with the help of an experienced fitter. Wearing a tight-fitting T-shirt or sweater when trying the different prostheses will enable you to get a good idea of their shape and how well they fit.

If you have had a partial mastectomy that has only slightly altered the size and shape of you breast, the breast care nurse will be able to augment it with a silicone shell, rather like a thin, scooped-out prosthesis. Alternatively, a small, light prosthesis can be stitched into your bra cup. Partial prostheses are also available in a range of sizes and shapes.

Costs of prostheses

In the UK, prostheses are supplied and fitted free of charge to women who have been treated under the National Health Service (NHS). They can be fitted by specially trained nurses, such as breast care nurses, hospital appliance officers and fitters from the manufacturers. Some fitters are men and you may like to check with the ward sister before your fitting if you would find this unacceptable.

If you are being treated privately, you will have to pay for your prosthesis and fitting, although some private health insurance schemes may contribute towards this cost.

Replacement prostheses

If you have been treated under the NHS, you can request a new prosthesis when your existing one begins to show signs of wear, is damaged, or if you gain or lose enough weight to make a significant difference in the size of your breasts.

Your breast care nurse will be able to arrange a fitting for you to choose a replacement. If your first prosthesis was fitted by an appliance fitter, contact the hospital appliance department for advice; you may need the authorization of your family doctor, consultant or breast care nurse, and the appliance fitter will be able to advise you about what to do.

Bras

Some under-wired bras put pressure on the silicone of a permanent prosthesis, which could cause it to split, but there are some breast forms available that can be worn with under-wired bras. Bras worn with prostheses should be able to hold the breast shape in place and prevent it slipping, but otherwise there is no other restriction on the type of bra you can wear.

Your breasts should be accurately measured and you should make sure that your bra fits well. At some large department stores there are staff experienced in fitting women following breast surgery.

If necessary, you can ask the breast care nurse or appliance officer about having a pocket fitted to a bra in which to insert your prosthesis. This service is usually available on the NHS in the UK.

Chapter 14

Breast reconstruction

Breast reconstruction is an option being taken up by increasing numbers of women following mastectomy. Although breast reconstruction can be undertaken for women with significant distortion or asymmetry of the breast following a wide local excision, it is usually unnecessary and the results are often unsatisfactory, in that the prosthesis has not been tailor-made for the cavity and may be extruded. For these reasons, most surgeons avoid breast reconstruction following wide local excision, and it should be carried out on only a very limited scale by a plastic surgeon.

Each of the techniques for breast reconstruction has its own merits and disadvantages and any one of several may be suitable for a particular woman. However, what is most appropriate for one woman may not be appropriate for another. It is therefore important that, before undergoing any type of breast reconstruction, you discuss your options with your reconstructive surgeon so that, between you, you can choose the most suitable one.

Breast reconstruction can involve using only tissue from another part of your own body or implanting an artificial prosthesis with or without the use of your own tissues.

Prosthetic reconstruction

Reconstruction of the breast with a prosthesis (implant) can usually be done immediately at the same time as a mastectomy by a breast surgeon, sometimes in collaboration with a plastic surgeon. In this case, it makes use of the existing mastectomy incision and very little additional operative time is required. Alternatively, it can be performed as a delayed procedure. However, reconstructing a breast to match a normal 'droopy' breast is difficult with a prosthesis alone.

The prosthesis itself consists of a silicone and/or polyurethane envelope that can be filled with various liquids (in the USA, almost always saline) or gels to mimic the consistency of normal breast tissue beneath the skin. Breast implants do not last forever and will eventually wear out, leading to leakage of the contents or rupture of the implant. If silicone gel leaks from the implant, it may cause a foreign-body tissue reaction resulting in a tender lump, and the prosthesis may need to be replaced.

Silicone implants

There is no scientific evidence to support the concerns people have had about the silicone in breast implants causing malignancy or autoimmune disease. However, the controversy about the long-term safety of silicone gel as a filling for breast implants has led to restrictions on its use in the USA. If you are worried about having a silicone implant, you should discuss with your reconstructive surgeon the advantages and disadvantages of each of the different fluid fillings before you make a decision.

If there is not enough skin remaining on your chest after a mastectomy to allow a prosthesis to be placed beneath it, skin may have to be imported from another part of your body (usually the back or upper abdomen) to create a space for the prosthesis (see below).

Tissue expansion

A possible alternative to importing skin is to expand the existing skin of the chest by inserting a special balloon under it, which is then gradually inflated with a salt solution (saline) over a period of weeks or months until the correct size of breast is achieved. Once the skin has been stretched sufficiently, the balloon can be removed and replaced by a soft, permanent prosthesis. To recreate the natural droop (ptosis) of the breast, the skin is over-expanded before the implant is inserted.

The process of tissue expansion may involve two operations, the first to insert the expander and fill it, and the second (after 6-8 weeks) to remove it and replace it with the definitive prosthesis. However, newer devices, such as the Becker prosthesis, enable the whole procedure to be undertaken during a single operation. These prostheses incorporate a central saline filling chamber and a silicone prosthesis. Once inserted, the amount of saline can be adjusted by means of valve, which is removed at a minor operation (usually involving only a local anaesthetic) when expansion of the breast is complete.

If your pectoralis major muscle is still intact (see p. 80), a tissue expander can be placed in a pocket underneath this muscle rather than directly under your skin. This helps to reduce the risk of complications occurring in the future, particularly for women who have had radiotherapy, which damages the blood vessels in the skin and may weaken it and make it more likely to allow protrusion of the breast prosthesis.

Although good cosmetic results can be obtained by tissue expansion, and an artificial nipple can be created with a skin graft (see below), it should be understood that, as with all methods of reconstruction, a perfect breast cannot be refashioned in this way.

Side-effects of prosthetic reconstruction

If an infection develops following prosthetic reconstruction, the implant may have to be removed, at least temporarily. Extrusion of the implant may occur if the skin has been weakened, for example by radiotherapy or an infection.

Although the body generally tolerates the foreign material of a prosthesis, a capsule of fibrous tissue forms around it. In some women, the fibrous tissue becomes thick and the capsule it has formed around the implant contracts, thus altering the shape of the prosthesis and causing a marked firming in the texture of the reconstructed breast. When this complication (known as capsular contracture) does occur, it is most likely to do so within the first year or two after the implant has been inserted, although it is possible many years later. The breast may become hard and painful and sometimes further surgery is necessary to regain the desired breast shape or to remove the implant.

Occasionally, particularly in young women, prostheses have to be removed because they are causing pain.

Other possible complications of prosthetic reconstruction include the implant moving from its original position, or leaking or deflating. Surgery may be necessary in these cases to reposition or replace the prosthesis.

Pedicled skin and muscle flaps

A pedicled flap is made by taking skin and muscle from another part of the body and placing it on the chest wall to replace the tissue removed during a mastectomy. The tissue transported to create a pedicled flap remains attached at some point - either via a section of the tissue itself or via blood vessels - to the site from which it is taken. As the tissue used to make the flap comes from the woman herself, this is sometimes known as autogenous tissue reconstruction.

A common procedure to create a flap following a mastectomy involves using the large muscle on the back (the latissimus dorsi muscle) and its overlying skin. A section of this muscle and skin is separated from the back, with some of its blood vessels still attached, and is then tunnelled beneath the skin to the front of the chest. If this skin and muscle alone are not enough to augment the chest to match the size of the other breast, a small prosthesis may be placed within the space created to provide symmetry.

This method of reconstruction is useful when tissue expansion is not possible, for example after radiotherapy or when a single-stage prosthetic reconstruction is required. In some cases, the extra muscle cover it provides for the prosthesis is also important.

Although the loss of part of the large muscle from the back does not usually have any significant functional effect, its removal leaves an obvious scar, which can stretch.

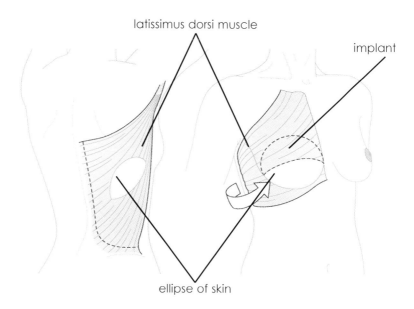

latissimus dorsi muscle

implant

ellipse of skin

Reconstruction of the breast using the latissimus dorsi muscle. *A section of the muscle and an ellipse of overlying skin are brought from the back and passed beneath the skin to the chest. If required, a breast implant can be placed in the space created.*

The imported skin will (to some degree) be a different colour from, and will therefore contrast with, your remaining breast skin, although this tends to improve with time.

Another type of autogenous tissue reconstruction involves the use of the rectus abdominis muscle (the 'six-pack' muscle) together with a large flap of overlying skin and subcutaneous tissue from the lower abdomen. (Once the skin has been removed from the lower abdomen, the navel is re-sited.) This is known as a transverse rectus abdominis myocutaneous (TRAM) flap. It is usually large enough to create a good-sized breast with natural droop and texture, and an artificial prosthesis is not required.

Removal of the excess abdominal tissue in this operation has an effect similar to that of a 'tummy tuck' operation, although the scar tends to be higher than in the cosmetic operation. It can occasionally leave the abdominal muscles weakened (although not usually significantly so),

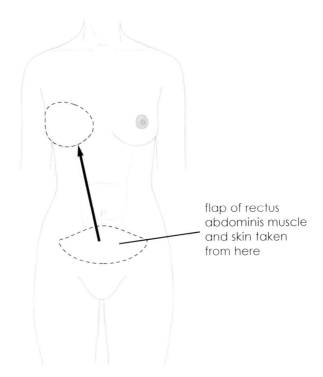

flap of rectus
abdominis muscle
and skin taken
from here

Reconstruction of the breast using the rectus abdominis muscle. *A flap of muscle and skin is taken from the lower abdomen, rotated, and tunnelled up beneath the skin to the chest. A breast implant is not normally necessary.*

which may be of significance if it leads to a tendency for a hernia to develop.

Some of the blood vessels remain attached to the skin and muscle as they are transposed from the abdomen to the chest. However, the normal blood supply to the skin is altered during this operation and consequently healing can be slow. Wound dressings may therefore be required for a week or two longer than normal. Occasionally, significant portions of the transferred tissue can die and further minor surgery may then be necessary to allow healing to take place.

Microvascular tissue transfer

Reconstruction of a breast using this technique involves transferring tissue from one site in the body (usually the lower abdomen), separating it from its normal blood supply and re-attaching it on the chest wall by microsurgery. Small sections of some blood vessels remain attached to the transferred tissue, and very fine surgical techniques are used, as well as high-powered magnification, to join the severed ends of these blood vessels to veins and arteries in the chest or axilla region.

This technique gives the best shape and most natural look of all the breast reconstructions. It may not involve the removal of any muscle from the abdomen, but, if it does, less is required than with the pedicled TRAM flap. Thus, as the blood supply is more secure, healing is usually quicker. However, the operation itself is complex and takes longer than the pedicled TRAM flap, thus involving a longer anaesthetic time. It may fail completely in up to 10% of cases and is most suited to young, fit women who do not smoke and are not obese.

Nipple reconstruction

Less than 50% of women undergoing breast reconstruction take up the option of nipple reconstruction. If you do wish to have nipple reconstruction, you will probably have to wait until your breast reconstruction has settled and the scars have softened, so that the position of the new nipple can be matched as nearly as possible to that of your other breast.

There are various techniques that can be used to create a nipple and areola. The nipple is usually reconstructed from local skin or from skin taken from the other nipple; the areola is formed from skin grafted from the groin area or from the other areola. Colour may be added to the areola by tattooing, and its irregularities beneath the skin can be simulated with cartilage grafts. However, with time, the projection of the nipple may be affected by natural changes and by the pressure from a bra. There is also often a difference in the colour of the areola when compared to that on the unaffected breast.

An alternative is to use an external nipple prosthesis, which can sometimes be held in place by suction rather than being attached with adhesive.

Timing of breast reconstruction

Most of the reconstructive procedures described above can be done at the same time as a mastectomy, although the more complex ones are usually best left to a later date, which may be anything from a few weeks to many years.

When reconstruction is undertaken will depend largely on the nature of the cancer, on the preferences of your surgeon and your own wishes, and on the availability of a reconstructive surgeon. Although some breast units can offer reconstruction, most depend on a close relationship with plastic surgeons.

It is important that you understand fully what is involved in breast reconstruction, and you will probably be given counselling before your operation to help you make an informed decision, particularly if it is going to be done at the same time as a mastectomy.

Surgery to the opposite breast

The aim of reconstructive surgery is to create a breast that matches the unaffected breast as nearly as possible, and this may sometimes only be achieved by performing additional surgery on the other breast. This additional surgery may be done at the same time as or after the reconstructive surgery. The decision as to when it is done will depend on various factors, which the surgeon should discuss with you. The advantage of surgery to the unaffected breast being done after reconstructive surgery is that it allows time for the reconstruction to settle.

An operation called reduction mammoplasty can be carried out to reduce the size of a large breast, but although this can result in a normal-looking breast with normal sensation, the resulting scars can be quite large. It is more common for a droopy breast to be uplifted by a technique known as mastopexy. Your reconstructive surgeon will be able to discuss these possibilities with you.

Chapter 15

Palliative care

For women whose breast cancer is incurable, there is now considerable care and support available from hospices and specially trained nurses based in hospitals, cancer centres and the community.

Care that cannot cure is called palliative, and there is a great deal that can be done to make living with cancer a less frightening and stressful experience for sufferers and their families. Palliative care is not just for people who are about to die; it is long-term care that can continue for months or years. Women can live full and happy lives with incurable breast cancer and many take advantage of the support that is available to improve their quality of life.

In the UK, hospice-based care and the support of Macmillan nurses (see below) are free to all who need them, being funded by charities and/or the National Health Service (NHS).

Hospices

If you have breast cancer that has spread to other parts of your body to such an extent that it is not curable, your family doctor, consultant or a specialist nurse such as a breast care nurse may suggest hospice involvement. Many people are shocked at this suggestion, because they imagine hospices to be places people go to die. However, although some people choose to spend their last days in a hospice, the main job of hospice staff is to support cancer patients, and their families, and to help them remain well and to live as full and normal a life as possible for as long as possible - which in many cases means continuing support for years.

Hospices have several aims:

❖ to help cancer patients live full and happy lives,

- to provide pain relief and to control any other symptoms of cancer that may arise,

- to counsel and support cancer patients and their families,

- to offer financial advice and information about grants and financial assistance that may be available,

- to provide regular home visits to support and care for cancer patients and their families and enable people to be cared for in their own homes rather than in hospitals,

- to provide education and courses on palliative care for nurses and doctors.

Some hospices also have in-patient facilities where people can go if they have symptoms that need to be brought under control, or simply to give their carers at home a week or two's respite. Many also have day-care facilities where cancer sufferers can spend the day involved in leisure activities such as painting, woodwork or making jewellery, where they can have their hair done, be bathed if this is becoming difficult at home, talk to a doctor or social worker, or just sit and chat in a friendly and supportive environment.

Specialist nurses based within hospices or in the community work closely with family doctors (who remain in overall charge of their patients' care) as well as with community nurses and social workers. Their special skills and experience enable them to co-ordinate the care their patients receive and to make sure they have the emotional support and medical treatment they require.

Some women prefer not to be referred to a hospice and some manage well alone, but many who do accept this help find their quality of life and ability to cope with their disease much improved.

Macmillan nurses

Macmillan Cancer Relief was set up in the UK in 1911 to provide care and support for cancer patients. This national charity now helps to improve the quality of life for cancer patients and their families at home, in hospitals and in special cancer units.

The charity has trained more than 2000 Macmillan nurses - all with at least 5 years' experience - who work in the community and in hospitals around Britain. It continues to fund these specially trained nurses for up to 3 years in posts in hospitals, after which the health authority takes over the financial responsibility.

Your family doctor or district nurse may suggest involving a Macmillan nurse to help with your care. Macmillan nurses play a role similar to that of hospice-based nurses, giving advice and emotional support to women and their families, and working closely with other medical professionals to advise about pain relief and symptom control as necessary. They are also involved in the training of doctors and nurses to help them develop the special skills required for the care of cancer patients and, with hospice staff, have been largely responsible for the increased awareness of other health professionals to the particular care these patients need.

Other treatment centres

The effects of complementary or alternative therapies are difficult to assess, in part because they are often only resorted to by people for whom conventional medicine has no more to offer in terms of cure.

There are private centres that advocate special non-medical therapies to help people 'fight' or live with cancer. Your family doctor, consultant or a specialist nurse should be able to give you details of any such centres in your area; alternatively, you can contact one of the associations listed in Appendix IV. Although, in the UK, the NHS does not fund alternative therapy centres, some have trust funds to help meet the costs for those who cannot afford them.

Appendix I
Questions and answers

The answers to most of these questions can be found elsewhere in this book. However, you may find them helpful in compiling your own list of points to raise with your doctor or breast care nurse. It is useful to write down questions as they occur to you, and to take your list with you to your doctor's appointment, as most people find it difficult to remember the things they wanted to ask when they are trying to take in the information being given to them by their doctor.

The answers given here are general, and your doctor or surgeon may have slightly different information to give you, depending on your own particular circumstances and on what happens at your hospital.

Do ask your family doctor, the hospital doctor who is in charge of your care, your breast care nurse or other member of the nursing staff if there is anything you do not understand. No question is too trivial, particularly if it concerns something that is worrying you.

1. While in the bath recently, I could feel a small lump in my breast, but a couple of days later it seemed to have disappeared. Should I do anything about it, or 'leave well alone'?
It is always better to seek your doctor's advice if you are concerned about a change in your breast. The breasts do tend to become lumpy before and during a menstrual period and it is therefore best to examine them 7 to 10 days after the start of a period. It could well be that what you felt was a normal cyclical change. However, do ask your doctor to examine you, to put your mind at rest and so that any necessary tests can be arranged.

2. I do not like feeling my breasts, but worry that by not doing so I am risking missing any small lump that could develop. Is there an alternative to this sort of breast examination?
Many women feel as you do, and the effective alternative is to examine your breasts regularly by looking at them. If you get used to their normal appearance, you should be able to detect any change, which may be a sign of something wrong. Look particularly at their shape, for any

discharge from the nipples, and any changes in the surface of the skin such as dimpling. Examining your breasts for any visible signs of disease can be done in the bath, shower or, for example, when applying deodorant.

3. A discharge has recently started to leak from one of my nipples. I am afraid to go to my doctor in case this is a sign of cancer. What should I do?
It is important that you make an appointment to see your doctor as soon as possible. Although there are various causes of nipple discharge, a bloodstained discharge could be (amongst other things) a sign of breast cancer, and the earlier this is treated the better. A milky or watery discharge could be caused by the use of a contraceptive pill or by recently stopping taking the pill. A greenish or yellowish discharge (which may be blood stained) could be due to a benign condition called duct ectasia, which can be treated by the surgical removal of the ducts just under the nipple. Another cause of a bloodstained discharge is a duct papilloma, a benign tumour that can be treated by an operation to remove the affected duct.

Your doctor will probably refer you to a consultant, who may want to arrange for you to have a mammogram to exclude cancer and to discover the reason for the discharge. If the cause is obviously benign, and the discharge is light, you may not need any further treatment: some women are happy to put up with a slight nipple discharge if they know it has no sinister implications.

4. I understand that, as I am now 65, I am no longer entitled to regular breast screening by mammography under the NHS. Will I have to pay for this to be done privately if I wish to continue with it?
Although you will no longer be called for 3-yearly breast screening, you are still entitled to continue it if you wish to do so. You can telephone your breast-screening clinic or mammography unit to make an appointment, or mention to your doctor that you would like to continue to have regular breast screening.

5. After a recent needle biopsy of a cyst in my breast, I have extensive bruising and tenderness in the area. Is this a sign of something wrong?
Bruising is caused by blood leaking from tiny blood vessels under the surface of the skin and is likely to occur to some degree following a biopsy,

whatever the precautions taken to prevent it. There is unlikely to be any cause for concern, and the bruising should gradually disappear over the next few days or weeks. If it does persist, is painful or spreads, ask your doctor's advice.

6. I have been referred to a general surgeon at my local hospital to investigate a lump in my breast. My family doctor said there is no specialist breast surgeon in our immediate area, but having thought about it again, I would rather see a breast specialist, even if it means travelling to do so. However, I am embarrassed about asking my doctor to change the arrangement. What should I do?

Almost all areas now offer specialist breast care and it is unlikely to be difficult for a referral to be arranged for you. It is, in fact, important that you *do* see a breast care specialist. A consultant who specializes in breast diseases will inevitably have more experience in this field than a general surgeon who does not have a specific interest in breast diseases. You may prefer to write to your doctor to request a referral to a breast specialist if you are anxious about talking to him or her again. Alternatively, you could contact your local hospital and ask if there is a breast care nurse you could talk to, as she may be able to advise you and to support your request for another referral. The charity Macmillan Cancer Relief will also be able to give you names of the breast specialists in your area.

7. Following the recent discovery of a small lump in my breast, an appointment has been made for me to see a specialist. I am 48 years old. What are the chances that the lump is cancer?

Although most types of breast cancer are more common in women around the time of menopause, approximately only 1 in 10 of those who are referred to a specialist with breast problems are found to have cancer. There are, of course, different types of breast cancer with different prognoses, but, in general, the outcome may be better if a small lump is treated at an early stage of development.

8. I frequently have pain in my breasts that does not seem to be related to my periods. I cannot feel a lump. What should I do, and what might be the cause of this pain?

Non-cyclical breast pain can have several causes, most of which are benign. It is not common for breast cancer to be associated with pain in the breast, although it can be. You should make an appointment to see your doctor, having first made sure that you are wearing a well-fitting bra.

If you have not been measured for a bra for some time, and particularly if you have lost or gained a significant amount of weight recently, it may be that the bras you wear are too big or too small and are not supporting your breasts properly. Breast pain that is not related to the menstrual periods can also be referred pain from a back or shoulder problem, and your doctor will probably want to investigate this possibility.

Sometimes, the cause of breast pain is never discovered, but it does often resolve itself in time.

9. I am 48, and have recently been able to feel hardness around the edges of both my breasts. What is this likely to be?

The breast tissue changes in women around the time of menopause, and what you are feeling is likely to be a benign condition called dysplasia or fibrocystic disease. However, it is essential to check with your doctor to rule out any other possible cause.

10. I am about to have a mastectomy. Will I need to wear special bras after my operation, and will I be able to wear swimsuits and sundresses?

There is no reason why you should need special bras; it is likely that the bras you usually wear can be adapted to hold and conceal a prosthesis. This is also likely to be true for most of your clothes. If there is a breast care nurse at your local hospital, do discuss this with her. Swimsuits, bras and sundresses can usually have a pocket sewn into them to hold the prosthesis, and this will allow you to take part in all sports and your usual activities without worrying about it becoming dislodged. Mastectomy swimsuits are available, but they are expensive, and should be unnecessary if your own can be adapted.

Although prostheses can be damaged by the under-wiring of strapless bras, it is probably all right to wear one for short periods of time if you want to wear a strapless dress. Low-cut dresses may not conceal your prosthesis, but, apart from this, there should be no restriction on the clothes you will be able to wear.

11. I am due to have a wide local excision within the next few days. How long does this operation last?

Most breast operations last about an hour, even mastectomies. You will therefore be under the anaesthetic for only a short period of time. Your operation is likely to be done as day-case surgery, so you should be able to return home once you have recovered from the anaesthetic.

12. How long will I have to be in hospital following my mastectomy?
Although the length of time spent in hospital varies depending, for example, on each hospital's normal practice and each woman's general state of health, it may only be 3 or 4 days before you are able to go home - at most about 8 to 10. Sometimes, mastectomies are done as day-case surgery, in which case you will be able to go home with your drain in place when you have recovered sufficiently from the anaesthetic. Psychosocial factors also play a part in the length of time some women spend in hospital.

13. I am very keen on gardening and want to know if I will be able to move my arm following my mastectomy, or whether I will always have restricted arm movement?
Although your arm movement may be restricted following your operation, you should be able to start to move your arm more easily within a few days. You will probably be advised about some gentle shoulder exercises to do after your mastectomy and, if you do these regularly, it will not be long before you can move your arm normally without any discomfort or stiffness. In due course, you will be able to do the gardening and all your other activities as normal. The sooner you start the shoulder exercises the better, but do not do so until you have been told by the medical staff that it is all right. Finger exercises can be done immediately after your operation.

14. The consultant has said that I should consider whether I would prefer to have a wide local excision or a mastectomy to remove a cancer from my breast. I do not want to make this decision myself, because I do not know enough about it, but I do feel that I should take the responsibility for choosing. What can I do?
Although most doctors now feel that patients should be able to take part in decision making, and some people prefer to make their own choices, it is perfectly acceptable to leave the final decision to your consultant. If you want more information, or a second opinion because you cannot decide what to do, then do ask for it. Your breast care nurse will be able to provide you with the information you require and to help you make the decision about which operation to have. She will also be able to tell you how to go about making an appointment with another consultant. Although

a second opinion is likely to be the same as the one you have already obtained, this in itself may put your mind at rest.

Most consultants will be quite prepared to do what they think best if you prefer not to have to make the decision yourself.

15. How long will I have to wait for the results of some tests to see if a lump I have in my breast is cancer?

In the UK, all women with a 'suspicious' breast lump are now seen at a 'one-stop clinic' within 2 weeks of referral. The results of the tests done at this appointment (and therefore the diagnosis) are almost always available on the same day. It is then normal for any necessary treatment to be started within 2 weeks of the clinic appointment.

16. I am very concerned about having treatment with the drug tamoxifen, because I have heard reports that it can cause cancer and has other serious side-effects. Is this true?

Tamoxifen has a variable effect on the menstrual periods, usually reducing them. It may cause the periods to cease altogether, but is not a reliable contraceptive, and occasionally causes erratic periods in pre-menopausal women. A post-menopausal woman who experiences bleeding should be referred to a gynaecologist for an investigative hysteroscopy.

The most commonly experienced side-effects of tamoxifen include weight gain, hot sweats and flushes, vaginal dryness and irritation and recurrent thrush. If the drug is taken for 10 years or more, there is also an increased incidence of dysplasia (irregularity of the endometrial cells) and possibly of endometrial cancer, which is why tamoxifen is given to women for no more than 5 years. However, most women feel that, as the drug is an effective treatment for the cancer they have, the very low risks are worth taking.

If you want more information about the available research into the use of tamoxifen, ask your consultant to discuss it fully with you before you start any treatment.

17. I have had a mastectomy and there does not seem to be any sign of spread of my breast cancer to other parts of my body. However, I am constantly anxious about any small ache or pain I have in case it is a sign of cancer in the bones or brain. Can I ask for a total body scan to reassure myself that there is no further cancer in my body?
Unfortunately, there is no test available that will confirm the presence or absence of cancer everywhere in the body. If you do develop any symptoms, tell your doctor, as scans can be done of individual parts of your body if necessary. Your doctor is likely to be sympathetic and understand your anxiety, and will be quite prepared to put your mind at rest about any specific symptoms.

However, even if it were possible to scan the whole body, any microscopic cancer cells that were present would not be visible, and the scan would therefore not tell you anything conclusive. The possibility that cancer could have spread before an operation to remove the breast, or that it could recur in the future, is well understood as a cause of anxiety to women who have had breast cancer, and you should receive all the support you require when trying to come to terms with this.

You will have regular check-ups for many years so that any symptoms or signs can be picked up early, but do talk to your family doctor, consultant or breast care nurse if you are worried, and do not be afraid that you are pestering them - they will understand your concerns.

18. What will the wound look like when I have had a mastectomy? I have a fear of seeing it after the operation and of being horribly disfigured for the rest of my life.
There will probably be a clear dressing on your wound after your operation to allow it to be inspected easily. This dressing will remain in place until your stitches are removed, or for up to 10 days if your wound has been stitched with an absorbable material. Through the clear dressing you will be able to see the cut edges of the wound and either a single 'running' stitch or separate stitches across the wound itself. The cut edges may be red and angry looking, and there is likely to be some bruising. Once your stitches have been removed or the wound has started to heal, it will begin to look much better.

Although many women find the first sight of their wound shocking, most do gradually get used to seeing it as it heals. Within a few months, it will probably have faded to a white or pinkish line, which will fade still further over the years.

As the mastectomy will remove your entire breast, you will be left with a flat chest wall on that side, and the wound may be a horizontal or diagonal line. Your nipple will also have been removed during the operation. Sometimes, however, there is still fat left on the chest that was overlying the breast. If so, you will have some breast contour rather than a dip where your breast used to be. There may be puckering around the wound, which may settle after a while.

Following a wide local excision, when the nipple is retained, there is usually some nipple distortion, particularly if the operation has been done to remove a tumour just beneath the nipple. The length of the scar will depend on the size of the lump that has been excised. Following a mastectomy, however, there should eventually be only a neat line where the skin was cut.

19. If I have to have chemotherapy or radiotherapy following my breast operation, what side-effects can I expect to experience?

The drugs used nowadays for chemotherapy are much improved in terms of their side-effects, and you may not experience any at all. It is unlikely that your hair will drop out and, although you may feel tired and nauseous for a while, many women do not even suffer these problems.

Radiotherapy for breast cancer is similarly unlikely to have any seriously debilitating side-effects, although (as with chemotherapy) different women react differently. The skin in the treated area may become sensitive, red and dry, and you will be advised about how to care for it during your treatment.

Do ask your consultant and/or breast care nurse to discuss any possible side-effects of the particular therapy you are to receive.

20. There is a breast care nurse at my local hospital, but as my breast problem is not cancer, would I be able to talk to her?

Breast care nurses should be able to give information and support to all women with breast problems, whether malignant or benign. Although their main responsibility is the care of women with breast cancer, they have experience with all types of breast diseases. Do telephone the breast care nurse and tell her about your problem; she will certainly be helpful and sympathetic, and will refer you to a more appropriate source of information if she is unable to help you herself.

21. I am due to have a mastectomy and have been told that it would be possible for breast reconstruction to be done at the same time. I am in my thirties, and think I would be happier with a permanent 'breast' rather than an external prosthesis. However, I am anxious about having to make this decision immediately. How can I obtain enough information to help me to decide?
Your consultant and breast care nurse should be able to give you the information you require. In the UK, Breast Cancer Care can also provide you with advice and information, and may be able to put you in touch with a local mastectomy support group so that you can talk to women who have been in the same situation.

It may be that your breast surgeon intends simply to insert an implant after removing your breast, but he or she should be happy to discuss the other possible options open to you, or you could ask to talk to a reconstructive surgeon if there is one in your area.

If you really cannot decide what to do - and it is a difficult decision to have to make at a time when you are already under stress - it may be better to have your mastectomy now and consider breast reconstruction at a later date, when you have had time to weigh up all the possibilities and their advantages and disadvantages.

Appendix II

Private care in the UK

There are various reasons why people choose to have their operations done privately. They may have private health insurance, be covered by a private health scheme run by the company for which they work, or they may be able to pay for private care themselves. Whatever your situation, you will not find that the standard of medical care you receive in a private hospital is any different from that available on the National Health Service (NHS). However, you may prefer the privacy of a private hospital, or you may find the much-reduced waiting time to see a consultant and the opportunity to enter hospital for your operation at the time of your choice are more convenient for you. If you have an operation in an NHS hospital, you may rarely see the consultant and may be examined and treated by different doctors in the consultant's 'firm'. At a private hospital, you will receive personal care from the consultant throughout your stay. The facilities at a private hospital are likely to be more like those of a good hotel and will certainly include a private bathroom.

The information given throughout this book is equally relevant whichever system you choose. This appendix deals with the aspects of private health care that differ from those of the NHS.

Private health insurance

If the company you work for has a private health insurance scheme, your Company Secretary will be able to give you details and should be able to tell you if the company insurance covers you for consultation with the surgeon and for your breast operation.

If you have your own private health insurance, the insurance company will be able to tell you exactly what is covered by your particular policy, if this is not clear from the literature you already have.

There are different levels of health insurance and you need to read your policy carefully to make sure you know which costs are covered. Most private hospitals have an administration officer who will check your policy for you if you are in any doubt. The members of staff at the hospital are likely to be very helpful and will try to sort out any problems and queries you have. However, do read your policy carefully, and any information sent to you by the hospital, as unexpected charges - such as consultants' fees that you thought were covered by your insurance policy - could add up to quite a lot of money.

It is essential that you inform your insurance company before embarking on any private treatment to make sure that all aspects of it are covered by your policy. You may need to ask the insurance company to let you know - in writing - whether your policy covers the cost of a prosthesis and its fitting if you are going to want one after your operation. This cost is not always included and can be quite high.

With some types of private health insurance, you will need to ask your family doctor to fill in a form stating that your operation is necessary and cannot be done in an NHS hospital within a certain time period due to long waiting lists. You will have to pay your doctor for this service, which will cost a few pounds. This money is not redeemable from your insurers.

Fixed Price Care

You may be in the position of being able to pay to have your operation done privately, in which case the Bookings Manager at a private hospital will be able to give you an idea of the cost involved. Some private hospitals run a service known as Fixed Price Care: a price can be quoted to you before you enter hospital that covers the cost of your operation and a variety of other hospitalization costs. You should always ask to have the quotation in writing before you enter hospital, with a written note of everything it covers. The fixed price you are quoted should include all the costs of your in-patient stay at the hospital, the operating theatre fees, any medication you require, and the fees for the surgeon, anaesthetist and pathologist - but do make sure that this is the case. Once you have a quotation, you should not have to worry about any hidden costs that you had not accounted for. However, in some cases, the price quoted to you by the hospital may not include the fees of the consultant surgeon or consultant anaesthetist and you may have to ask your surgeon for a note of these.

With Fixed Price Care, all the hospitalization costs included by that particular hospital are covered should you need to stay longer than expected in hospital (usually up to a maximum of 28 days) as a direct result of complications arising from your original reason for admission. In other words, if you develop some problem while in hospital that is unrelated to the breast problem that led to your need for an operation, the price you have been quoted will not cover treatment to deal with this. If, on the other hand, you develop a complication as a direct result of the breast disorder or of the operation to treat it and your consultant decides to keep you in hospital for longer than originally planned, all the costs that arise from your stay and are included in the hospital's fixed price (again, with the possible exception of consultants' fees) will be covered. At some hospitals, the quoted price will also cover your treatment should you have to be re-admitted due to a complication related to your original operation and arising within a limited period of time after your original discharge.

The only extra charges that you will have to pay to the hospital will probably include those for telephone calls, any alcohol you have with your meals, food provided for your visitors, personal laundry done by the hospital, hairdressing and for any similar items such as you would have to pay for in a hotel. It is usually possible for a visitor to eat meals with you in your room and for tea and snacks to be ordered for visitors during the day. (You will also have to pay these extra charges before you leave the hospital if you are being treated under private health insurance.)

It is important, therefore, that you ask in advance for written confirmation of the price you will have to pay for your stay in hospital and what is included in the quotation. If the hospital does not have a Fixed Price Care or similar system, make sure that all potential costs are listed.

Arranging the operation

Although the medical treatment you receive in a private hospital will be similar to that available at any NHS hospital, there are some basic differences between the two systems.

As with the NHS, you will have to be referred to see a consultant privately by your family doctor. Most doctors have contacts with particular consultants (and private hospitals) to whom they tend to refer patients. If there is a private hospital you particularly want to go to, or a consultant you have some reason to prefer, you can ask your doctor to make an appointment for you. Do be sure that an appointment is made for you to see a *breast specialist*. You can check this yourself by finding out what type of NHS practice a particular surgeon runs.

After the visit to your doctor, you are unlikely to have to wait longer than a week or two before you see the consultant at an out-patient appointment. Your appointment may be at the private hospital where your operation is to be carried out, at an NHS hospital that has private wards, or at the consultant's private consulting rooms. Once the decision has been made to go ahead with surgery, you will probably be able to enter hospital at your convenience within another week or two.

You will receive confirmation of the date of your operation from the Bookings Manager of the hospital you are to attend. You will probably also be sent leaflets and any further relevant details of how to prepare for your admission to hospital. Do read these carefully, as knowing how your particular hospital organizes things will help you to be prepared when you arrive for your operation. You will be sent a pre-admission form to fill in and take with you when you are admitted.

If your operation is being paid for by insurance, you will be asked to take a completed insurance form with you when you are admitted to hospital. You should have been given some of these forms when you first took out your policy, but your insurance company will be able to supply the correct form if you have any problems. If you are covered by company insurance, the form will probably be filled in and given to you by your Company Secretary.

Admission to hospital

When you arrive at the hospital, the receptionist will contact the admissions department and a ward receptionist will come to collect you. If you are paying for your stay in hospital yourself, you will probably be asked to pay your bill in advance at this stage if you have not already done so. Otherwise, you will be asked for your completed insurance form. The ward receptionist will take you to your room (probably a single or double room) and show you the facilities available there. You are likely to have a private bathroom, a television and a telephone by your bed. The ward receptionist will explain hospital procedures to you and will leave you to settle in.

A member of the nursing staff will then come to make a note of your medical details, in much the same way as described in Chapter 7. The main difference you are likely to notice if you have been treated in an NHS hospital before is that this time there is much less waiting for all the routine hospital procedures to be dealt with. The nurse to patient ratio is higher in private hospitals and so someone is usually available to deal with the pre-operative procedures quite quickly.

Your consultant will deal with your medical care throughout your stay, will visit you before the operation, perform the operation (with the assistance of the anaesthetist and the operating staff) and visit you again when you are back in your own room. Trainees - whether doctors or nurses - do not work in private hospitals. The consultants are responsible for their own patients and supervise their care themselves. Most private hospitals now have resident medical officers - fully qualified, registered doctors who are available 24 hours a day to deal with any emergencies that may arise.

Preparing for your operation

When visiting you on the ward before your operation, the consultant will mark the side and site of your breast lump. When the time for your operation approaches, a porter and nurse will take you from your room to the anaesthetic room. In many private hospitals, you will not be moved from your bed onto a trolley until you have been anaesthetized; the bed itself will be wheeled from your room. Similarly, you will be transferred back from the trolley to your own bed in the recovery room while you are still asleep. You therefore go to sleep and wake up in your own hospital bed.

Your operation will be performed in the same way as described in Chapter 9. When you are fully awake, you will be taken back to your room to rest.

Discharge from hospital

When you are ready to be discharged from hospital, the ward receptionist will ask you to pay any outstanding charges not covered by the hospitalization charge. You will be given any medical items you may need from the hospital pharmacy.

Adjuvant therapy

Although adjuvant treatments for breast diseases, such as radiotherapy and chemotherapy, can be undertaken in private care, not all private hospitals have the facilities to carry these out. For example, very few can offer on-site radiotherapy, and this treatment is likely to be given at an NHS centre.

Differences and similarities

The main aim of the staff of any private hospital is the same as that in an NHS hospital - to make your stay as pleasant and as comfortable as possible. Because the staffing ratio is higher in private hospitals, more emphasis can be placed on privacy and comfort.

The consultant surgeons and anaesthetists almost always work in an NHS hospital as well as in a private hospital, so you will receive the same expertise and skill under both systems. However, in an NHS hospital you may not actually be operated on by the consultant surgeon who heads the surgical team and, indeed, you may not see the consultant at all during your stay.

Private hospitals arrange their operating lists differently from NHS hospitals. The NHS hospitals have 'sessional bookings' for their operating theatres. This means a particular day is set aside at regular intervals for a specialist in one type of surgery to perform operations. In private hospitals, the consultants can book the use of an operating theatre (and the assistance of the staff who work in it) on any day, at any time that suits them. Therefore, your operation can take place privately with minimum delay and at a time that is convenient to you and your consultant.

It is also possible, even if you are already on an NHS waiting list, to tell your family doctor or consultant at any time that you would like to change to private care. If the consultant you have already seen under the NHS does not have a private practice, you can ask to be put in touch with one who can see you privately.

Although some private hospitals may have their own breast care nurses, the majority do not. However, if you would like to talk to a breast care nurse, the hospital should be able to arrange this. Bearing in mind how important the role of these specialist nurses is now recognized to be, it may be a good idea to request this service. The same applies to counselling services, which will probably be made available if you request them.

Summary

There are several reasons why, if they can, some women choose to have their operations done privately, paid for either by private health insurance or from their own pockets. Some find it much more convenient to be able to have a say in when their operation is to take place. The NHS, under which the majority of people are treated, naturally has longer waiting lists. If time is an important factor for you, you may be happy to pay to have your operation done at a time that you find convenient.

Some people simply prefer the smaller, more intimate setting they are likely to find in a private hospital. Private hospitals rarely deal with accidents and emergency treatment; the operations carried out in them are normally planned, at least a day or two in advance. Therefore, they do not have the bustle of an NHS hospital, which has to deal with emergency admissions as well as the routine admissions for non-emergency operations.

Appendix III

Medical terms

Abscess An infected, pus-filled swelling containing debris from disintegrating tissue.

Adair's operation An operation to remove ducts from under the areola of the breast which is performed to treat duct ectasia. It is also known as Hadfield's operation.

Adjuvant therapy Treatment that is helpful to, or whose effect is maximized by combination with, another form of treatment but that alone may not comprise a complete therapy.

Admission letter The letter sent to patients giving details of their hospital admission.

Adrenalectomy An operation to remove both the adrenal glands that can lead to regression of recurrent breast cancer in some cases. The adrenal glands are tiny glands above the kidneys that produce various hormones, including oestrogen-like hormones that can stimulate tumour growth in some types of breast cancer. Adrenalectomy is no longer commonly performed.

Allergy An over-sensitivity to a substance that causes the body to react against it. The allergic reaction can be mild, such as an itchy rash, or more severe, possibly involving fainting, vomiting or loss of consciousness. You should make sure your doctor knows of any allergies you may have so that they can be noted in your medical records.

Alveolus A small sac-like pocket (or gland). Alveoli develop at the ends of the breast ducts at puberty, enlarge during pregnancy, and secrete droplets of milk in lactation.

Anaesthesia The absence of sensation.

Anaesthetic A drug used to cause loss of sensation in part of the body.

Anaesthetist A highly trained doctor who is skilled in the administration of anaesthetics.

Analgesic A drug that blocks the sensation of pain; a painkiller.

Anastrozole (Arimidex) A type of drug called an aromatase inhibitor. It is sometimes used as hormone therapy to treat breast cancer and acts by interfering with the production of the sex hormones in the ovary and adrenal glands.

Antibiotic A substance that kills germs (bacteria).

Anticoagulant A substance that prevents the blood from forming clots (coagulating), for example heparin.

Anti-embolism stockings Stockings worn by patients during their operations and while they are immobile post-operatively. The stockings assist the circulation of blood in the legs and help to prevent blood clots forming.

Anti-emetic A drug that helps to combat feelings of sickness.

Areola The pigmented part of the breast.

Autogenous tissue reconstruction Reconstruction of a breast using tissue from the woman's body. The reconstruction can be in the form of a pedicled flap, or can be done by microsurgical transfer of tissue to the breast.

Axilla The armpit.

Benign Non-malignant; a benign disease is one from which recovery is likely following adequate treatment. Benign tumours remain localized at the site at which they developed (i.e. they do not spread), and have no harmful effect other than possibly squashing adjacent organs and therefore interfering with their functioning.

Biopsy The surgical removal of a small piece of tissue from a living body for examination under a microscope for the purposes of diagnosis.

Breast awareness Examination of the breasts to detect any apparent changes that occur and that might indicate disease. Women may visually inspect or manually examine their breasts (breast self-examination).

Breast care nurse An experienced nurse who specializes in caring for women who have breast conditions - both malignant and benign.

Breast mouse A colloquial name for a fibroadenoma, so called because it is a very mobile lump, which slips out of the fingers when an attempt is made to grasp it.

Breast screening The examination of women's breasts by mammography (X-rays). It is carried out every 3 years in the UK for women between the ages of 50 and 65. Breast screening is done in an attempt to detect changes in the breasts - particularly cancer - which may occur most commonly in this age group and which are most easily seen in the breasts of older women.

Bromocriptine A drug that is sometimes used in the UK to treat cyclical breast pain when no other treatment has been effective. It can cause side-effects such as fluid retention and headaches. More serious problems have been reported in the USA, as a result of which it is no longer used there.

Cancer A malignant growth caused by the uncontrolled multiplication of cells. If left untreated, it will eventually invade nearby areas of the body and spread to distant parts.

Cannula A very fine tube or needle that is inserted into a vein, usually in the back of the hand. Fluids can be introduced into or removed from the body via the cannula, and drugs can be administered through it for anaesthesia during an operation. Cannulas are usually made of plastic, but used to be metal or glass.

Capsular contracture A complication that can follow insertion of a breast implant and that involves tightening of the capsule of fibrous tissue which forms around it. The reconstructed breast becomes firm to the touch or, in severe cases, hard and painful.

Carcinoma A cancer that occurs in epithelial, glandular, tissue and that can spread locally and to other parts of the body. Carcinomas are always malignant, but can vary in severity.

Carcinoma in-situ A carcinoma that remains in the site at which it first developed. This is a pre-malignant condition.

Cautery/Cauterization A process used to stop bleeding using a high-frequency electric current. The heated tip of an instrument is placed at the end of a blood vessel to seal it.

Chemotherapy Treatment with drugs, such as for cancer.

CMF A combination of the cytotoxic (anti-cancer) drugs cyclo-phosphamide, methotrexate and fluorouracil, which is often used in chemotherapy for breast cancer.

Complication A condition that occurs as the result of another disease or condition. It may also be an unwanted side-effect of treatment.

Consent form A form that patients must sign before surgery to confirm that they understand what is involved in their operation and during the anaesthesia they are to have, and that they give their consent for the operation to take place and for the doctors to undertake any procedures that they feel to be necessary.

Conservative treatment Treatment carried out to effect a cure that avoids the use of drastic measures.

Consultant An experienced and fully trained doctor who specializes in a particular type of medicine.

Cosmetic scar A scar that is not easily apparent once it heals, and that is achieved, for example, by stitching the wound under the surface of the skin (subcuticular closure).

Cyclical breast pain Breast pain that is associated with the menstrual cycle.

Cyclogest A form of the sex hormone progesterone that is sometimes used to treat severe period-related (cyclical) breast pain.

Cyst A fluid-filled swelling. Cysts can develop anywhere in the body as smooth, hard, sometimes painful lumps.

Cystic carcinoma A rare but serious form of ductal breast cancer.

Cytological examination The examination of cells under a microscope for the purposes of diagnosis.

Danazol A drug that is sometimes used to treat cyclical breast pain. Because of its side-effects, including fluid retention and headaches, it is usually given as a last resort if no other treatment is effective.

Day-case surgery An operation carried out on a patient who is in hospital for one day only, with no overnight stay.

Deep vein thrombosis (DVT) A blood clot that forms in the deep veins of the body, most commonly in the calf of the leg.

Diagnosis The identification of a disease based on its symptoms and signs.

Differentiation (of tumours) The identification of the types of cells involved in a tumour, which can have an effect on the likely outcome of the disease. The closer the resemblance of a tumour to its cells of origin, the better the outcome is likely to be.

Discharge letter The letter given to patients as they leave hospital for them to deliver to their doctor's surgery. The letter informs the doctor of any relevant details about the patient's operation and any follow-up that is needed.

Dissection The separation of structures within the body for identification or during surgery.

Ductal cancer Cancer arising within the ducts of the breast. The ductal cancers are the most common type of breast cancer.

Duct ectasia A benign condition involving dilatation of the ducts beneath the nipple, which fill up with their own secretions.

Duct papilloma A benign tumour of the epithelium that lines the body's surface and most of its hollow structures, such as the ducts within the breast. Papillomas can form in breast ducts near the areola.

Dysplasia The abnormal development of tissue or change in a tissue type.

Eczema Inflammation of the skin causing itching or burning.

Electrocardiogram (ECG) The activity of the heart recorded as a series of electrical wave patterns.

Electrocautery Cautery involving the use of an instrument whose tip is heated by an electrical current.

Embolus A blood clot or air bubble that has broken off and can pass through the blood vessels causing sudden blockage.

Endometrial cancer Cancer of the endometrial lining of the womb (uterus).

Evening primrose oil A substance found by some women to be effective in relieving cyclical breast pain, the active ingredient of which is also available as gamma linoleic acid. Although studies have proved its efficacy, there is still controversy about its use amongst some medical professionals. Some women also find it helpful in relieving non-cyclical breast pain.

Excision Removal of a part by cutting it away.

FEC A combination of the cytotoxic (anti-cancer) drugs fluorouracil, epirubicin and cisplatin, which is often used in chemotherapy to treat breast cancer.

Fibroadenoma A solid, benign tumour of fibrous and glandular tissue in the breast that is surrounded by a capsule. Because fibroadenomas are mobile, they are colloquially referred to as 'breast mice'.

Fibroadenosis Also known as hyperplastic cystic disease or benign mammary dysplasia, this is a general, benign condition involving lumps and cysts in the breast. It is most common in women between the ages of 35 and 50.

Fine-needle aspiration biopsy The use of a thin needle to remove a small sample of cells from a lump for cytological examination under a microscope.

Fixed Price Care The system used by some private hospitals in the UK whereby a fixed price is quoted for a particular type of operation and some of the hospitalization costs associated with it.

General anaesthetic A drug that induces sleep and abolishes the sensation of pain in all parts of the body.

Genetic predisposition The likelihood of a person to develop a particular disease dependent on their genetic make-up. Some diseases are more likely to develop in people whose close relatives (who have similar genes) have had it. For example, some types of breast cancer are more likely to affect women whose grandmothers, mothers, sisters or aunts have suffered from it.

Gland An organ that produces substances such as enzymes and hormones.

Goserelin (Zoladex) A drug that is sometimes used as hormone therapy for breast cancer. It is given as a monthly injection to inhibit the pituitary stimulation of the ovaries and induces a temporary menopause. The menstrual periods resume when treatment stops.

Gynaecomastia The condition in which a man develops one or two breasts.

Hadfield's operation Another name for Adair's operation to treat duct ectasia.

Haematoma A blood-filled swelling that can develop following surgery if a blood vessel continues to bleed. If the blood is spread within the tissues, it appears as a bruise.

Haemorrhage Bleeding; the escape of blood from arteries or veins in any part of the body.

Heparin A substance produced naturally within the body that helps to prevent the blood from clotting. It is also given by injection before and after surgery to people who are at high risk of developing blood clots, for example those who have suffered a previous deep vein thrombosis.

Histological examination The examination of a small sample of tissue that has been taken from the body by biopsy.

Hormone replacement therapy (HRT) Treatment with hormones that is given to women as their levels of oestrogen and progesterone fall before and after menopause. HRT is now considered an important means of combating the risk of brittle bones, which can cause serious problems in elderly women.

Hypophysectomy An operation to remove the pituitary gland from the brain. The pituitary produces hormones that stimulate tumour growth, and this operation is carried out in an attempt to stop these hormones being produced, and thus control the growth of a tumour. Hypophysectomy is no longer advocated for treating breast cancer.

Incision A cut or wound made by a sharp instrument, such as during an operation.

Induction agent A drug used during anaesthesia to bring on sleep.

Infective 'mastitis' Inflammation of the breast caused by micro-organisms, which may be transferred through a cracked nipple via the hands, an infection passed from baby to mother while breast-feeding, a blood-borne infection, or infection resulting from a blocked duct containing stagnant milk in a lactating woman. The condition may respond to treatment with antibiotics, but often progresses to become a breast abscess.

Inflammatory carcinoma A rapidly growing ductal breast cancer that can resemble a breast abscess.

Inhalational anaesthetic An anaesthetic given as a mixture of gases that is inhaled through a facemask.

Intravenous anaesthetic An anaesthetic that is injected into a vein via a cannula, usually inserted into the back of the hand.

Invasion The spread of malignant cells via the blood or lymphatic fluid.

Inverted nipple A nipple that has turned inwards into the breast. Some women's nipples develop in this way, but sometimes an inverted nipple is a sign of breast disease.

Lactation The secretion of milk before and after childbirth.

Lactiferous duct A duct within the breast that receives milk from the secreting alveoli (lobules).

Langer's line A natural crease line in the skin. Some incisions for breast operations can be made along one of these lines so that the resulting scar is almost invisible.

Lobular cancer Cancer of the breast that develops within the lobules, often of both breasts. Lobular tumours are less common than the ductal forms of cancer.

Lobule A subdivision of a part in the breast that secretes milk.

Local anaesthetic An anaesthetic that numbs the area of the body around which it is injected.

Lymph The pale-coloured fluid that flows within the lymphatic vessels of the body and that contains disease-fighting cells called lymphocytes.

Lymph node Another name for a lymph gland into which lymphatic vessels drain.

Lymphocyte One type of white blood cell that is involved in fighting disease within the body.

Lymphoedema A condition in which lymphatic drainage is impaired and lymph collects in a part of the body causing swelling, tightness of the skin and pain.

Maintenance agent A drug used during anaesthesia to maintain the state of sleep.

Malignant Used to describe a tumour that is likely to spread locally and to distant parts of the body - a cancer. Malignant tumours invade the surrounding tissue and can spread to other sites within the body forming secondary tumours (metastases).

Mammillary fistula A condition involving discharge via the nipple and from the scar of an incision made, for example, to drain and remove an abscess in the breast. A connection persists between the nipple and the scar.

Mammogram An X-ray of the breast.

Mammography The study of the breast by means of an X-ray of the soft tissues.

Mammotome® needle A special needle with a vacuum device attached that is used in some types of breast biopsy to remove a sample of 6-12 cores of tissue for histological examination.

Mastalgia Pain in the breast, often occurring before a period but sometimes a sign of a minor or occasionally a more serious breast disease.

Mastectomy Complete surgical removal of the breast, and usually of the lymph nodes in the armpit.

Mastitis Inflammation of the breast.

Mastopexy Surgery to raise a drooping breast.

Medical history The record of someone's past health, including diseases, operations, allergies etc.

Medullary carcinoma An old-fashioned name given to a type of ductal tumour that is the 'least malignant' of the common ductal breast cancers. It is also known as lymphocytic or encephaloid carcinoma.

Megestrol (Megace) A drug that is sometimes used in hormone therapy to treat breast cancer. It is a progestogen - a synthetic form of the naturally occurring hormone progesterone.

Menopause The time in a woman's life when her menstrual periods cease. It signals the end of her reproductive ability and may be associated with troublesome symptoms.

Menstruation The discharge of blood from the lining of the womb that occurs through the vagina approximately monthly throughout a woman's reproductive life, except during pregnancy and lactation.

Metastases Secondary tumours that are at a site (or sites) distant from the original cancer.

Metastasis The spread of cancerous cells, through the blood or lymphatic vessels, from the site of the original tumour.

Metastasize To spread to a distant part.

Microdochectomy An operation to remove a duct from underneath the nipple that contains a warty growth (papilloma) or an early cancer. A probe is inserted into the affected duct and then surgically excised through a radial incision made from the tip of the nipple, taking with it the duct and the growth it contains as well as a small amount of breast tissue.

Microvascular flap A block of tissue attached to sections of an identified artery and vein that have been divided and then re-attached to blood vessels elsewhere in the body.

Microvascular surgery The rejoining of small (1-2 mm diameter) blood vessels using high-powered magnification and very fine surgical instruments and sutures.

Microvascular tissue transfer The transfer of tissue (usually from the lower abdomen) by microsurgical techniques to reconstruct a breast.

Modified radical mastectomy (Patey) An operation to remove the entire breast, all the axillary lymph nodes, and the smaller of the two chest muscles.

Monitoring device Equipment that is used to watch over the various activities of the body, such as the heart rate, pulse etc.

Nausea A feeling of sickness.

Neoplasm Any new formation of tissue; a tumour.

Nerve block An anaesthetic that is injected to cause loss of sensation in the nerves in a particular area.

Nil by mouth A term used to mean that no food or drink should be swallowed in the hours before an operation.

Nipple The projection from the areola of the breast on which the lactiferous ducts open.

Nipple discharge Fluid leaking from the nipple; it is usually benign and due to hormonal changes. However, it can be a sign of serious breast disease, particularly if blood stained.

Node sampling The excision of the lowest axillary lymph glands (nodes) so that they can be examined to give an indication of how far a cancer has spread.

Non-palpable Not able to be felt by touch.

Obesity An excessive amount of fat in the body. This term is non-specific and its use is being replaced by a figure calculated from height and weight measurements, known as the body mass index.

Oedema Swelling caused by the increased leakage of fluid from the blood capillaries that accumulates in the spaces between tissues.

Oestrogen A steroid hormone; in women, it stimulates sexual development at puberty and causes changes in the lining of the womb during the menstrual cycle. Oestrogens are produced by the ovarian follicle and by the adrenal glands situated above the kidneys.

Oncology The study and management of new growths; the study of cancer.

Oophorectomy The surgical removal of an ovary.

Ovarian cancer A serious form of cancer that develops in the ovary.

Paget's disease A quite serious but rare breast disease that resembles eczema but spreads slowly over the areola and may eventually destroy the nipple. Because this condition is caused by a cancer arising in a duct beneath the nipple, treatment may involve complete removal of the breast.

Palliative Something used to alleviate symptoms without being able to cure the condition that causes them.

Palpable Able to be felt by touch.

Palpation Physical examination using the hands.

Papillary carcinoma A rare variant of a non-specific ductal tumour that has a good prognosis. A bloody discharge from the nipple may be the first sign of this cancer.

Papilloma A benign, stalked tumour of the epithelium.

Partial mastectomy Also known as segmentectomy or wide local excision, this operation involves the removal of a quadrant of the breast including the tumour it contains and a wedge of normal surrounding tissue. Lymph nodes may also be removed from the armpit, and the operation is often followed by radiotherapy.

Peau d'orange Pitting of the skin that resembles the surface of an orange and that may be a sign of serious breast disease. It occurs when lymph vessels become blocked and fluid accumulates within the breast.

Pectoralis major muscle A large muscle that lies beneath the breast and forms the anterior wall of the armpit.

Pectoralis minor muscle A triangular muscle that lies beneath the pectoralis major.

Pedicled flap A block of tissue that has been transferred from elsewhere in the body but that retains some of its original attachments.

Peri-areolar incision An incision made around the pigmented areola to allow access to the ducts behind the nipple and to a centrally located breast lump.

Peripheral breast abscess A pus-filled swelling at the edge of the breast that is most common during lactation. Antibiotic treatment may be effective, but surgical incision and drainage of the abscess may be necessary.

Pituitary gland A gland situated in the brain that secretes various hormones.

Placebo An inactive substance that is given instead of a drug during pharmacological trials.

Plasma cell mastitis Inflammation of the breast due to ductal secretions produced in duct ectasia leaking out of the ducts and triggering a defence reaction by the body. A green, yellow or sometimes bloody nipple discharge may result, as may peri-areolar abscesses.

Post-menopausal After the menopause.

Post-operative Following an operation.

Pre-admission form A form that is sent out to patients before they enter hospital for an operation. The form contains questions about various aspects of the patient's medical history.

Pre-clerking admission procedure A procedure adopted by some hospitals whereby patients are asked to visit the hospital before an operation so that it can be explained to them, and they can ask any questions. Any necessary pre-operative tests, such as a blood test, are done at this appointment so that the results are available when the patient is admitted for surgery.

Pre-medication ('Pre-med.') Any drug that is given before another drug, for example one given an hour or two before an operation to relax the patient before anaesthesia is started.

Pre-menopausal Before the menopause; between puberty and the menopause.

Pre-operative Before an operation.

Pressure dressing A wound covering that exerts pressure and helps to stop bleeding.

Progesterone A steroid hormone that stimulates changes in the female reproductive organs, preparing them for pregnancy.

Prognosis An opinion on the probable course and final outcome of a disease that is made when all the known facts are considered.

Prognostication A forecast of the probable course and outcome of a disease.

Prolactin A hormone produced in the pituitary gland in the brain that stimulates milk production.

Prosthesis An artificial part, e.g. a leg, arm or breast.

Prosthetic reconstruction Surgery to reconstruct a breast using an artificial implant.

Ptosis Drooping of an organ. This is a natural feature of the breasts.

Pulmonary embolism A blood clot or air bubble that blocks the blood vessels in the lungs.

Pus A liquid produced as a result of inflammation and infection that contains both dead and living tissue fragments, cells and bacteria.

Pyrexia A fever.

Radical mastectomy An uncommon operation to remove the entire breast, the axillary lymph nodes, and the muscles of the chest wall.

Radical treatment Aggressive treatment aimed at curing a serious illness.

Radiotherapy Treatment with radiation.

Recovery room A ward near the operating theatre to which patients are taken after surgery so that they can be closely watched while they recover from the anaesthetic.

Recurrence The reappearance of symptoms or signs of a disease after a period of apparent recovery.

Reduction mammoplasty Surgery to reduce the size of the breast. It can be undertaken to match an unaffected breast to a reconstructed one.

Regression The disappearance of the symptoms and signs of a disease.

Retracted nipple A nipple that is drawn inwards to below the surface of the skin. A retracted nipple may be an early sign of breast cancer, but can also occur during breast development, when it has no sinister implications.

Risk factor Something that increases the chances of a particular person developing a particular condition. Risk factors include attributes that are already present, such as genes inherited from other members of one's family, or can be acquired, such as smoking.

Sarcoma A malignant tumour of connective tissue. Sarcomas in the breast are very rare.

Secondary tumour A tumour that develops at a site distant from that of the original, primary, tumour; a metastasis.

Segmental quadrantectomy A modification of a wide local excision to remove a breast lump and a segment of surrounding normal tissue.

Segmentectomy Another name for a partial mastectomy, an operation to remove a segment of the breast that contains a tumour as well as a wedge of normal tissue from around it. Some axillary lymph nodes may also be removed for staging purposes.

Self-examination (of the breasts) The examination of the breasts by feeling them all over with the flat part of the ends of the fingers in order to detect any physical changes such as lumps within the breast tissue.

Sentinel node The lowermost axillary lymph node, which is sometimes biopsied to determine whether breast cancer has spread to the lymphatics.

Seroma A collection of body fluids, such as blood and lymph, which can develop following an operation despite the use of drains. A persistent seroma can be treated by drawing off the fluid with a needle - a painless procedure.

Serratus anterior muscle The chest muscle attached to the upper ribs and shoulder blade, which is partially overlain by the breast.

Sign Something a doctor looks for as an indication of disease, such as a lump in the breast.

Simple total mastectomy Surgical removal of the entire breast, including the part which extends into the armpit, and some or all of the axillary lymph nodes.

Staging (of cancer) Classification of the development of a disease or condition. Staging of breast cancer is based on factors such as the size of the tumour, what type of cells it contains, and the amount it has spread. In some cases, the stage at which a cancer is discovered can have a bearing on the likely outcome of its treatment.

Step-down ward A ward to which day-case patients are taken in some hospitals to recover before going home after surgery.

Stereotactic core biopsy A recent modification of the core biopsy technique. A computer guides a Mammotome® needle to a non-palpable breast lump that has been located by mammography, and a single sample of 6-12 cores of tissue is removed for histological examination.

Sternum The breast bone.

Sub-areolar breast abscess A pus-filled swelling near the nipple that is often associated with nipple abnormality or plasma cell mastitis. Treatment with antibiotics or surgical excision and drainage of the abscess may be necessary.

Sub-areolar incision An incision made at the junction of the pigmented area and the rest of the skin of the breast.

Subcutaneous Under the skin.

Subcuticular Under the upper layer of the skin.

Sub-mammary incision An incision made in the crease underneath the breast to remove the breast completely but leave the skin and nipple intact.

Super-radical mastectomy Surgical removal of the breast, muscle tissue, the axillary and other lymph nodes.

Supraclavicular Above the collarbone.

Suture A surgical stitch or row of stitches.

Symptom Something experienced by a patient that indicates a disturbance of normal body function, for example pain or nausea.

Tamoxifen A drug used in hormone therapy for breast cancer that blocks the action of the female hormone oestrogen on the cancer cells, thus preventing their continued growth. Tamoxifen is usually given in the form of tablets.

Taxanes A group of drugs - including paclitaxel (Taxol) and docetaxel (Taxotere) - that are currently being assessed in clinical trials for the treatment of breast cancer.

Thrombo-embolic deterrent stockings (TEDS) Anti-embolism stockings that are worn by patients during operations and while they remain immobile to help prevent blood clots forming in the deep veins of the legs.

Thrombosis The coagulation of blood within a vein or artery that produces a blood clot.

Thrombus A blood clot that forms in, and remains in, a blood vessel or the heart.

Tissue expansion Stretching of the existing skin on the chest wall following a mastectomy so that an implant can be inserted to reconstruct the breast.

Transverse abdominis myocutaneous (TRAM) flap A flap of skin and muscle taken from the lower abdomen to reconstruct a breast.

Trastuzumab (Herceptin) A drug that is currently being assessed in clinical trials for the treatment of breast cancer.

Tru-Cut® biopsy The removal of a small core of tissue using a special Tru-Cut® needle. It is done in the breast to remove tissue from a suspicious lump so that it can be examined under a microscope.

Tumour A swelling, which can be benign or malignant. A benign tumour remains localized and does not spread to other parts of the body. It has no harmful effect other than to squash adjacent organs as it enlarges. A malignant tumour - a cancer - will invade the surrounding tissues, thus interfering with their normal functioning. Cells from malignant tumours can spread to other parts of the body by metastasis to form secondary tumours.

Ulcer A lesion of the skin in which the surface layers have been destroyed, exposing the deeper tissues.

Ultrasonography/Ultrasound Examination of the soft tissues of the body that involves the passage of high-frequency sound waves. The waves are reflected back from any solid object, much like an echo. Once processed by a computer, the sound waves can be used to build up a picture, which will delineate areas of tissue such as cysts or tumours.

Warfarin A drug taken orally to help prevent clots forming in the blood vessels; an anticoagulant.

Wedge excision The surgical removal of a segment of tissue.

Wide local excision An operation to remove a lump (usually malignant) together with a margin of normal tissue from around it.

Appendix IV

Useful organizations

Every country has its own organizations and societies that can provide information and advice about breast and other types of cancer as well as about benign breast conditions and problems such as lymphoedema that may result from treatment. The organizations listed alphabetically below are just a few of those in the UK. Because space is limited, only one address for each of the other main English-speaking countries is given at the end of the list. These are all good starting points for anyone seeking further information - both women themselves and health professionals - and many also have details of local and national support groups.

If you have access to the Internet, you will be able to find websites for these and other organizations throughout the world, some of which have links to local groups. If you have any problems, try typing 'breast cancer' in the 'Question' or 'Search' section on a general information site such as www.askjeeves.co.uk or www.google.com.

Breast Cancer Care
Kiln House
210 New King's Road
London SW6 4NZ
Telephone: 020 7384 2984
Helpline: 0808 800 6000
Website: www.breastcancercare.org.uk
Provides support and information to women affected by breast cancer as well as details of local self-help groups. All volunteers have personal experience of breast cancer and are trained to offer emotional support and practical advice.

Breast Care Campaign
Blythe Hall
100 Blythe Road
London W14 0HB
Telephone: 020 7371 1510
Website: www.breastcare.co.uk
Launched in 1991 to assist women with *benign* breast disorders, it provides information and advice about all types of breast condition.

CancerBACUP
3 Bath Place
Rivington Street
London EC2A 3JR
Telephone: 020 7696 9003
Helpline: 0800 800 1234
Website: www.cancerbacup.org.uk
A cancer information service that was set up as a charity in 1985 by a doctor following her own experiences of cancer. Various booklets are available free of charge to cancer patients and their families. A team of experienced cancer nurses will answer enquiries made by telephone or letter, and this should also be a good starting point for women who want details of cancer help organizations in their area.

Cancer Care Society
11 The Cornmarket
Romsey
Hampshire SO51 8GB
Telephone: 01794 830300
Website: details can be found on www.netdoctor.co.uk
Provides free confidential counselling, practical advice and an information library for people whose lives have been affected by cancer and can put people in touch with other cancer sufferers for mutual support. Advice on complementary therapies and respite breaks at holiday accommodation are also available.

Carers' National Association
20-25 Glasshouse Yard
London EC1A 4JT
Telephone: 020 7490 8818

3rd Floor, 162 Buchanan Street
Glasgow G11 2LL
Telephone: 0141 333 9494

11 Lower Crescent
Belfast BT7 1NR
Telephone: 028 9043 9843

Helpline: 0808 808 7777
Websites: details can be found on www.netdoctor.co.uk.
There are also sites for people in Northern Ireland (www.carersni.org) and in Scotland (available through www.show.scot.nhs.uk).
Provides support and information for carers throughout the UK. Various free leaflets are available at the 120 local branches.

CRUSE Bereavement Care

Cruse House
126 Sheen Road
Richmond
Surrey TW9 1UR
Telephone: 202 8939 9530
Helpline: 0870 167 1677
Website: www.crusebereavementcare.org.uk
Offers practical advice, counselling and support through its many local branches to anyone bereaved by death.

Disabled Living Foundation

380-384 Harrow Road
London W9 2HU
Telephone: 020 7289 6111
Helpline: 0845 130 9177
Website: www.dlf.org.uk
Provides information and advice about a variety of aids, which may be useful to people suffering from *lymphoedema* of the arm who have difficulty with everyday tasks such as opening jars, writing etc.

Institute of Complementary Medicine

PO Box 194
London SE16 7QZ
Telephone: 020 7237 5165
Website: www.icmedicine.co.uk
Useful for anyone wanting details of reliable practitioners of various kinds of complementary medicine or information about support groups.

Irish Cancer Society
5 Northumberland Road
Dublin 4
Telephone: 1 2310 500
Helpline: 1 800 200 700
Action Breast Cancer: 1 800 309040
Website: www.irishcancer.ie
The helpline is staffed by fully qualified nurses who are trained in cancer care. It can provide information on all aspects of cancer as well as details of support groups for women who have had a mastectomy. The society also funds home care and rehabilitation programmes run by voluntary groups. Night nursing in people's homes can be arranged when requested by a doctor or public health nurse.

Lymphoedema Support Network
St Luke's Crypt
Sydney Street
London SW3 6NH
Telephone: 020 7351 0990
Information Support Line: 020 7351 4480
Website: www.lymphoedema.org
Provides support, advice and information about treatment for people with lymphoedema and is involved in support groups throughout the UK.

Macmillan Cancer Relief
89 Albert Embankment
London SE1 7UQ
Telephone: 020 7840 7841

9 Castle Terrace
Edinburgh EH1 2DP
Telephone: 0131 229 3276

82 Eglantine Avenue
Belfast BT9 6EU
Telephone: 02890 661166

Lloyds Bank Chambers
33 High Street, Cowbridge
South Glamorgan CF71 7AE
Telephone: 01446 775679

CancerLine: 0808 808 2020
Website: www.macmillan.org.uk
A national charity that supports and develops a variety of services for people with cancer and their families, including Macmillan nurses.

Marie Curie Cancer Care

89 Albert Embankment
London SE1 7TP
Telephone: 020 7599 7777
Website: www.mariecurie.org.uk
Centres throughout the UK provide nursing care for cancer patients. The Marie Curie Community Nursing Service can offer home nursing (free of charge to patients) at the discretion of the local health authority. Welfare grant schemes are also available, which can be applied for through the district nursing service.

Tak Tent Cancer Support - Scotland

Flat 5
30 Shelley Court
Gartnavel Complex
Glasgow G12 0YN
Website: www.taktent.org.uk
Provides emotional support, counselling and information about cancer and its treatment. There are support groups throughout Scotland, and a counselling service is available at the centre. It also runs courses for cancer patients and their families.

The Ulster Cancer Foundation

40-42 Eglantine Avenue
Belfast BT9 6DX
Telephone: 028 9066 3281
Helpline: 0800 783 3339
Website: www.ulstercancer.org
Helps patients and their families cope with cancer, offering counselling, support and a fitting service.

Women's Nationwide Cancer Control Campaign
1st Floor
Charity House
14-15 Perseverance Works
London E2 8DD
Telephone: 020 7729 4688
Website: details can be found on www.netdoctor.co.uk
Founded in 1965, the aim of this organization is to promote the prevention and early detection of breast cancer. It provides information and advice about screening.

American Cancer Society
Telephone: 1 800 ACS 2345
Website: www.cancer.org

Australian Cancer Society
Level 4
70 William Street
GPO Box 4708
Sydney
New South Wales 2001
Telephone: 61 2 9380 9022
Cancer Information Service: 13 11 20
Website: www.cancer.org.au

Canadian Cancer Society
National Office
Suite 200
10 Alcorn Avenue
Toronto
Ontario MDV 3BI
Telephone: 416 961 7223
Website: www.cancer.ca

Cancer Society of New Zealand
PO Box 10847
Wellington
Telephone: 64 4 494 7270
Website: www.cancernz.org.nz